Natalie Cascella is the CEO and founder of Nuworld Botanicals and author of *Nuworld Botanicals DIY Raw Skincare Recipes*. Natalie has spent the last decade successfully growing her natural skincare brand by selling into major retail stores like Whole Foods Market.

Natalie has a business degree in marketing and has spent the majority of her career working for Fortune 500 companies before leaving her corporate life in 2015 to pursue entrepreneurship full time.

Her flagship retail store is located in downtown Oakville Ontario, Canada and features a unique concept in DIY natural skincare making. Her mission today is to teach natural skincare making and empower people of all ages to take control of the ingredients in their skincare. Natalie can be found teaching DIY skincare classes at her Oakville store and online, and coaching aspiring skincare entrepreneurs at her Masterclass.

Natalie Cascella

Nuworld Botanicals™

DIY Raw Skincare Recipes 2

From Our Store to Your Kitchen!

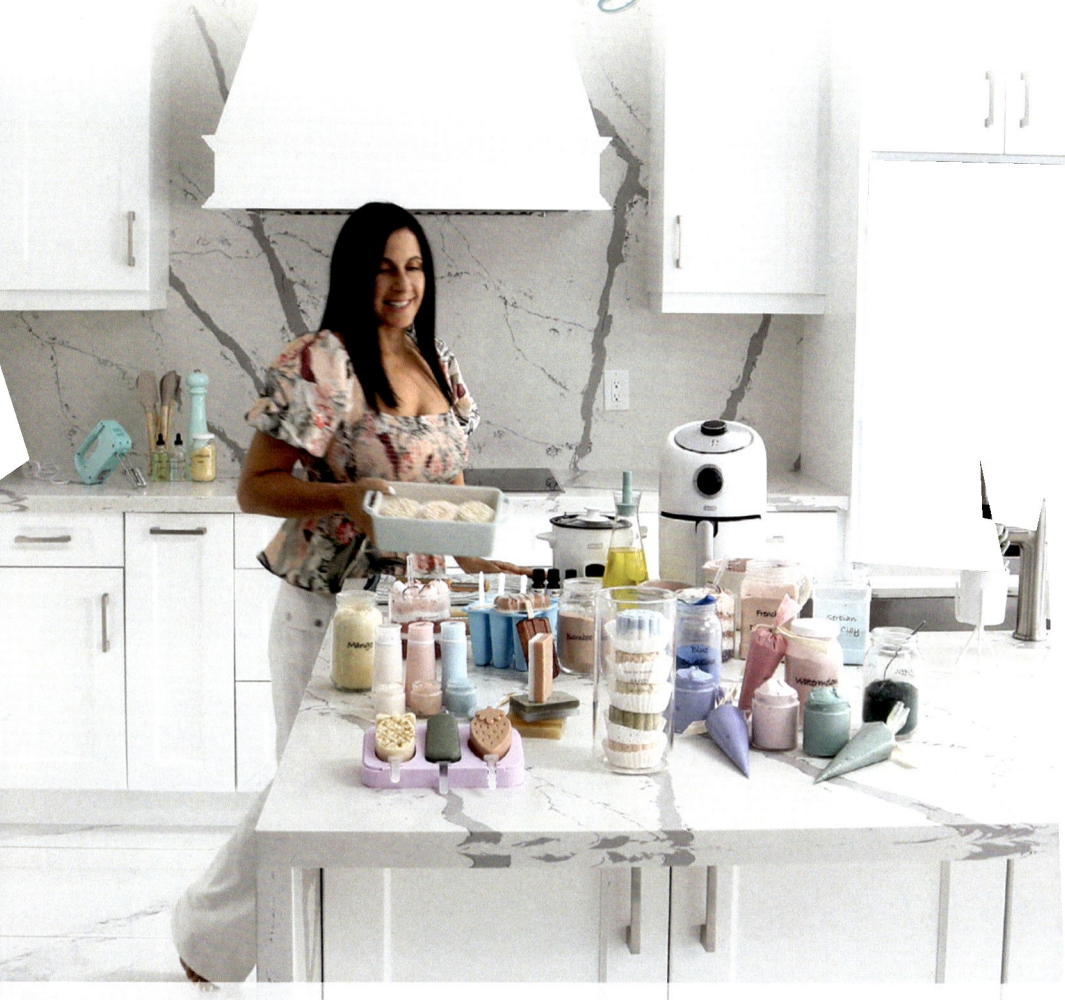

Quick and Easy Superfood Recipes

AUSTIN MACAULEY PUBLISHERS®
LONDON · CAMBRIDGE · NEW YORK · SHARJAH

Copyright © Natalie Cascella 2025

All rights reserved. No part of this publication may be reproduced, distributed, or transmitted in any form or by any means, including photocopying, recording, or other electronic or mechanical methods, without the prior written permission of the publisher, except in the case of brief quotations embodied in critical reviews and certain other non-commercial uses permitted by copyright law. For permission requests, write to the publisher.

Any person who commits any unauthorized act in relation to this publication may be liable to criminal prosecution and civil claims for damages.

Ordering Information
Quantity sales: Special discounts are available on quantity purchases by corporations, associations, and others. For details, contact the publisher at the address below.

Publisher's Cataloging-in-Publication data
Cascella, Natalie
Nuworld Botanicals DIY Raw Skincare Recipes 2

ISBN 9781685625221 (Paperback)
ISBN 9781685625238 (ePub e-book)

Library of Congress Control Number: 2021901176

www.austinmacauley.com/us

First Published 2025
Austin Macauley Publishers LLC
40 Wall Street, 33rd Floor, Suite 3302
New York, NY 10005
USA

mail-usa@austinmacauley.com
+1 (646) 5125767

To all of those hard-working artisan skincare makers making a positive impact on our skin, health, and the environment.

My husband, Johnny, and our children, Nick and Adrianna, for supporting me in pursuit of my dream business ten years ago and in writing this book. Lana Marconi, R.Ac., my sister and TCM acupuncturist (Marconi Acupuncture), for sharing her knowledge in health and wellness and inspiring my journey. My parents, Larry and Elisa, for their encouragement and igniting my entrepreneurial spirit. My incredible team of Master Mixologists, I want to acknowledge your assistance in creating this book, from the recipe trials and tests to the photography and product modelling, you guys rock! Linda, my graphic designer, there is no way I would have accomplished the feat of completing this book without your skills and expertise. Julius, for your invaluable contribution and visual media expertise. My publisher, the entire team at Austin Macauley Publishers, I am forever grateful for this opportunity you have given me, it means the world.

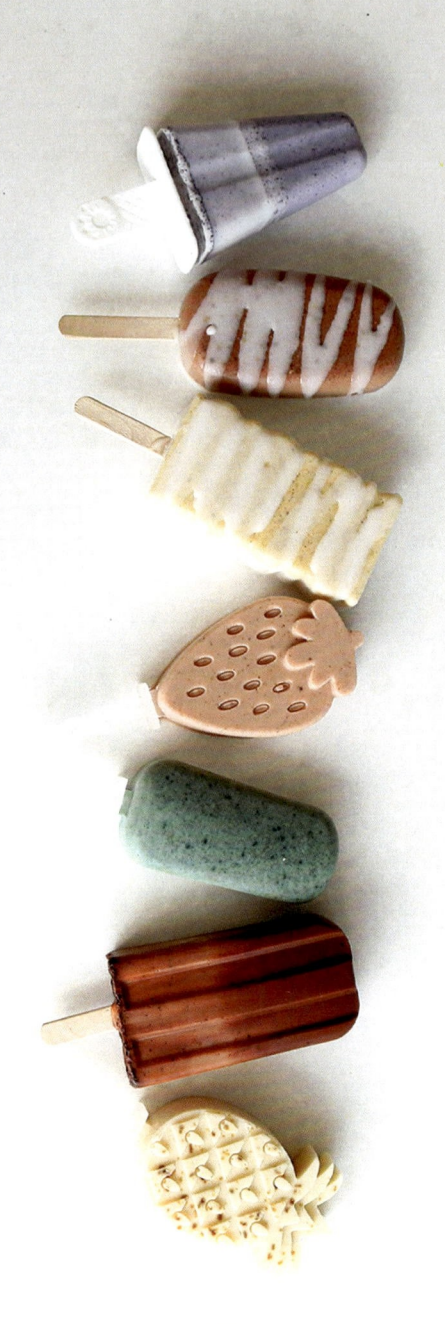

Contents

Hi there, DIY skincare makers!—8

Diy Kitchenware—10
Modern essentials for DIY cooking, baking and prepping recipes

How-to Guide—16
Guide to Superfood Bronzer Shades, Streamlining your DIY Pantry, Superfood Colour Guide, Natural Source Alpha-Hydroxy Acids and Vitamins, The Easy Melt and Pour Soap Method

At-Home Self-care Skincare Rituals—52
Build a Skincare Ritual, Facial Massage Rituals, Bath Rituals, Shower Rituals, Haircare Rituals, Lip Care Rituals, Bedtime Rituals, Guest Amenities

Diy Superfood Skincare Recipes—68
Salicylic Blueberry Face Wash, Vitamin C Creamy Exfoliating Cleanser, Mango Melting Milk Cleanser Balm, Lactic Apple Hydrating Mask, Salicylic Purple Potato Acne Mask, Glycolic Papaya-C Face Mask, Citric Tangerine-C Exfoliator, Vitamin K-Apricot Dark Circle Face Oil, HA-Hydrating Green Veggie Face Serum, Glycolic Fruits Hyperpigmentation Face Oil, Pineapple-Enzyme Sleep Cream, Retinol-A Golden Berry Face Cream, Lactic Coconut-Collagen Eye Cream, HA Banana Balm, Lactic Acid Apple Sleep Lip Mask, Butterfly Pea Lip Plump + Scrub, Sweet Dreams Aromatherapy Roll-on

Diy Superfood Bodycare Recipes—104
Cocoa-Coffee Toning Soapsicle, Blue Spirulina Soapsicle, Coconut Milk & Honey Waffle Hand Soaps, Power Berry Soapsicle, Banaba Leaf Magnesium Soapsicle, Turmeric-Pineapple Glow Soapsicle, Strawberry Vitamin C Soapsicle, Superfood Whipped Body Cream, Wolfberry Mineral Bath Soak, Pumpkin Mineral Bath Soak, Vitamin C Body Oil, Lemongrass Loofah Shower Oil, Blue Coconut Milk Bath, Avocado Superfood Balm, Baked Potato Shower Melts, Press n' Bake Superfood Bath Bomb, Raspberry Body Scrub

Diy Raw Haircare Recipes—140
Honey Humectant Hair Conditioner, Raspberry Repair Protein Treatment, Sky Blue Clay Hair Mask, Green Clay Scalp and Shower Bar, Yellow Clay Scalp and Shower Bar, Pink Clay Scalp and Shower Bar, Papaya Scalp and Body Scrub, Sweet Potato Scalp and Body Scrub, Broccoli Scalp Serum Treatment

Diy Superfood Bronzer Recipes—160
Pink Watermelon Highlighting Powder, Golden Pumpkin Bronzer, Cranberry-Copper Bronzer, Plum Potato Bronzer, Cocoa-Bamboo Bronzer, Bronze-Nude Lip Luminizer, Blush-Pink Lip Luminizer

Hi there, DIY skincare makers!

My name is Natalie and I'm the founder and CEO of Nuworld Botanicals. I've been making and selling my own natural skincare products for over a decade now. My big break came when I landed my products on the shelves of Whole Food Market stores. After successfully selling into major retail stores for 7-plus years I wanted this second book to reflect what my customers, students and readers wanted to see more of, so here we go:

More Skin-Boosting Superfood Recipes: If you've ever been to my store it's like a fresh smoothie bar, but for your skin! Like many of you, I use superfood powders at home in just about everything from cooking and baking to making smoothies. Superfood powders are chock-full of antioxidants and vitamins that deliver amazing results to our skin and they add beautiful natural colouring. Just check out my Superfood Colour Guide for product design inspiration.

Guide to Natural Source Skincare Acids: Yes there are chemical-free ways to get your skincare alpha-hydroxy acids and vitamins. Check out my handy How-to Guide for helpful pro-tips and DIY tricks.

Simple Kitchen Cooking & Baking Tools: I love using simple kitchen tools. I think you'll love my new bath bomb drying technique, and of course you know I use a rice cooker to melt everything I make. You don't need any specialized equipment to make any of my recipes.

Easy and Fast Soap Recipes: Melt and pour soap is the only type of soap making for me! It's quick, easy, 100% safe and effective. Check out our new superfood soapsicle creations, from pineapple bars to cocoa fudgesicles and go bananas with your own creations.

Home Self-Care Rituals: Our homes are an extension of our well-being and self-care at home is an extension of that. My hope is that you'll not only make these recipes but use them mindfully in your everyday self-care skincare routines.
Remember to take time out for yourself each day.

I can't wait for you to try these recipes for yourself!

Natalie

CREATE, BAKE AND DECORATE

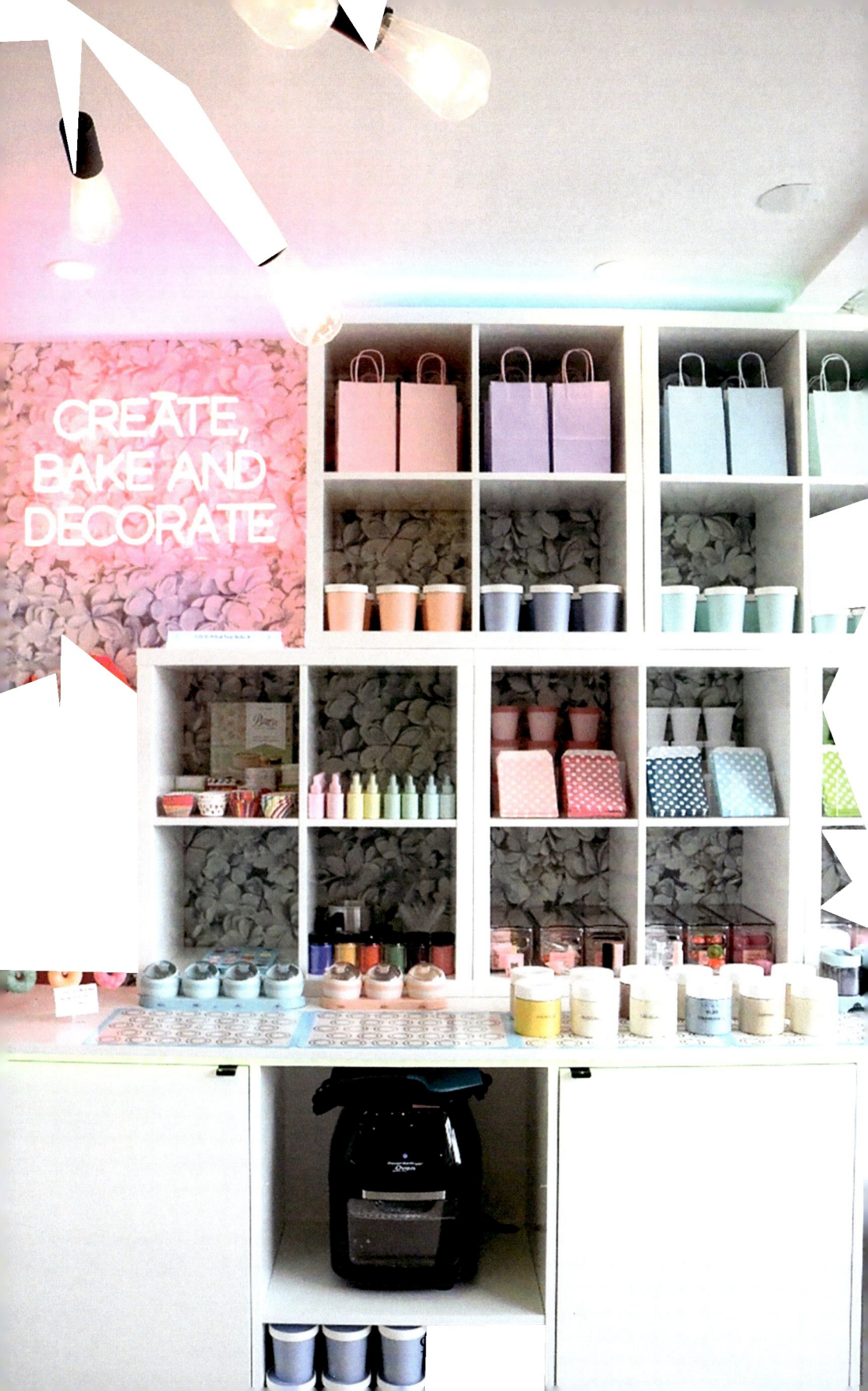

PIPE DREAMS

Piping bags aren't just for cake decorating! I like to put my superfood body creams in here and finish each jar off with a pastry-like swirl. Presentation is everything!

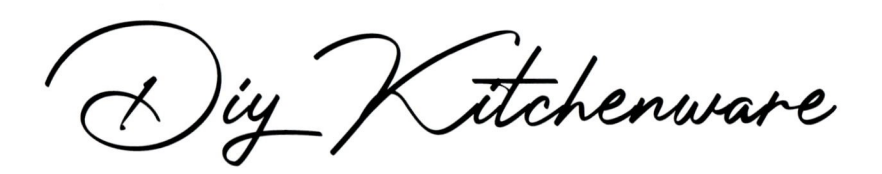

Diy Kitchenware

Modern Cookware | Bakeware | Prep Tools

COOK IT: DOUBLE BOILER HACK

My mini rice cooker by Dash® doubles as my double-boiler! It's perfect for experimenting with single-serving portions of soap, balms and more. Because it's portable, I can move it around my kitchen space. One pot does it all!

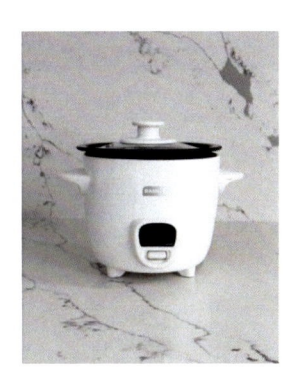

BAKE IT: AIR FRIED BATH BOMBS

Sure you can air dry your Bath Bombs— but that can take up to 24 hours! My new technique is to bake them dry. I simply pop them into my Air Fryer to dehydrate at 170°F for about 10 minutes and they're ready to be packaged up and/or used.

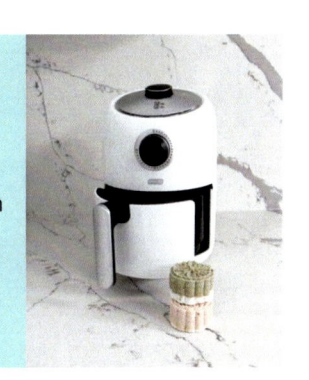

PRESS AND RELEASE

I love using this DIY bath bomb mold. It comes with interchangeable stamps, so you can create unique designs. Pack it with your mixture, place the mold on a flat surface, and press down to release your bath bomb.

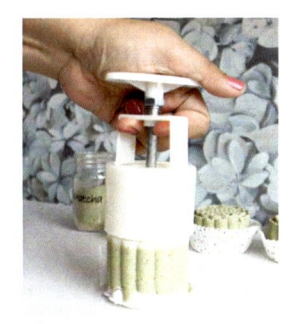

FRESH OLIVE OIL

At home, I'll decant cold-pressed organic carrier oils (like jojoba, apricot kernel and olive oil) in this air tight glass oil bottle dispenser. It's drip-free. Keeps my skincare oils fresh and my counter looking stylish too. Being that it's clear, it also helps me keep track of inventory.

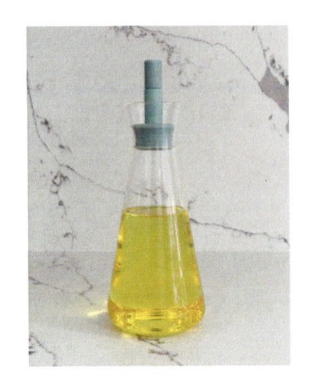

COLOUR PALETTE TEA TOWELS + OVEN MITTS

Since I'm working with an Air Fryer now, I need to keep my hands protected. I love these waffle-weave oven mitts and kitchen tea towels, they match my colour palette perfectly. The perfect addition to any DIY kitchen.

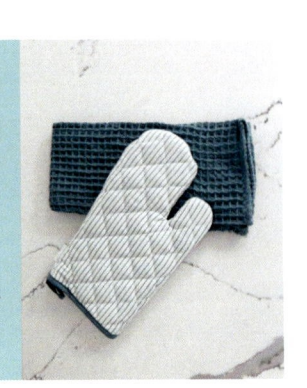

COMPACT SERVE n' BAKEWARE

This contemporary stoneware dish is the perfect size (and colour) for baking and serving yummy superfood bath bombs. Oven safe of course.

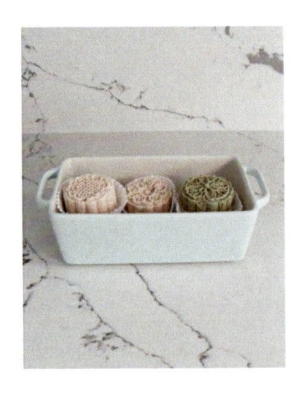

PERFECTLY SIZED PREP BOWLS

These mini preparation bowls are the perfect size for pre-portioning ingredients like waxes, exfoliants, extracts and butters. They also act as pinch pots, or dessert dishes.

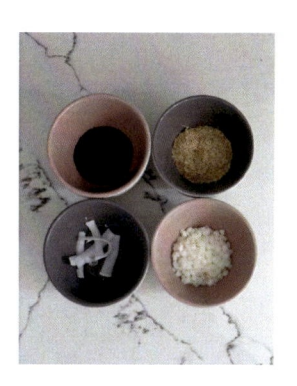

ELECTRIC BLUE

Creamy recipes come together quickly with the electric hand mixer. After my creams, conditioners, balms and butters have set in the fridge, I'll fluff them up with a handy electric mixer.

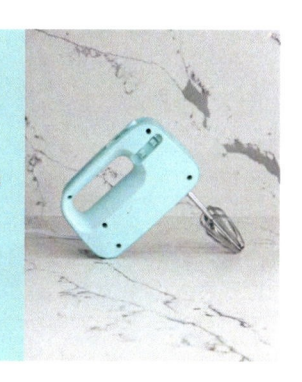

KITCHEN MEASURING BOWL

I love this dual purpose jug. Not only do I use it for taking measurements but it's wide enough for my balloon whisk so I can whisk up powder bronzers, clay masks and fluff up light creams. It's by Mason Cash.

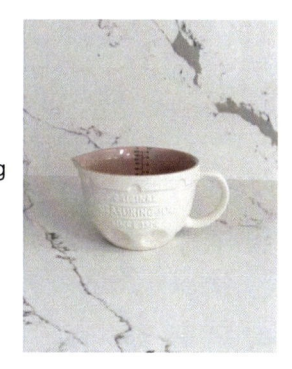

SPATULA ESSENTIALS

For perfect results and efficient prep work, I use a variety of silicone spatulas. Effective for getting every last bit of cream from the bowl and for stirring mixes. And these look super cute on my kitchen counter too.

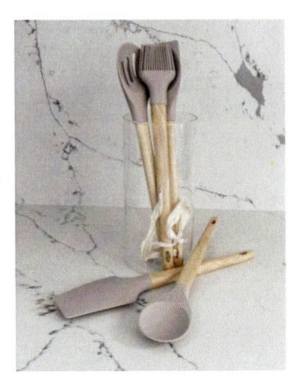

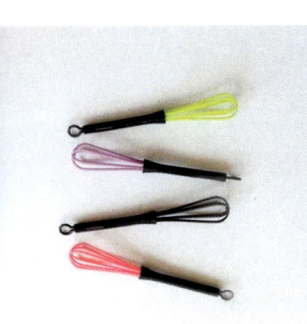

EVERYDAY BALLOON WHISK

What's the secret to fold dry ingredients into light-weight creams? Mixing clays and powders? Breaking down mineral salt chunks? It's all in the whisk!

I use two types of whisks: A stainless steel balloon whisk (on the right) and French whisks (on the left), which are perfect for small whipping tasks. The cute colours put some pep in my whip too!

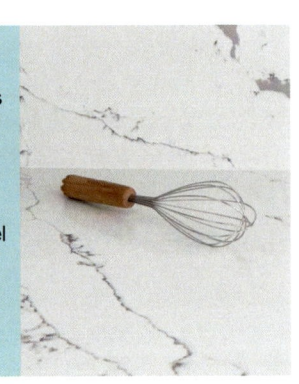

PRETTY SILICONE SHAPES

Silicone molds are perfect for soap making. They're super easy to clean and the product pops right out without breaking. These molds come in all types of shapes, sizes and colours. Just think outside the box (or mold) and you'll find what you're looking for.

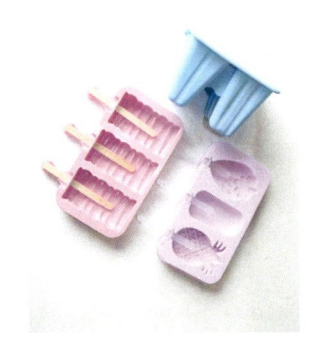

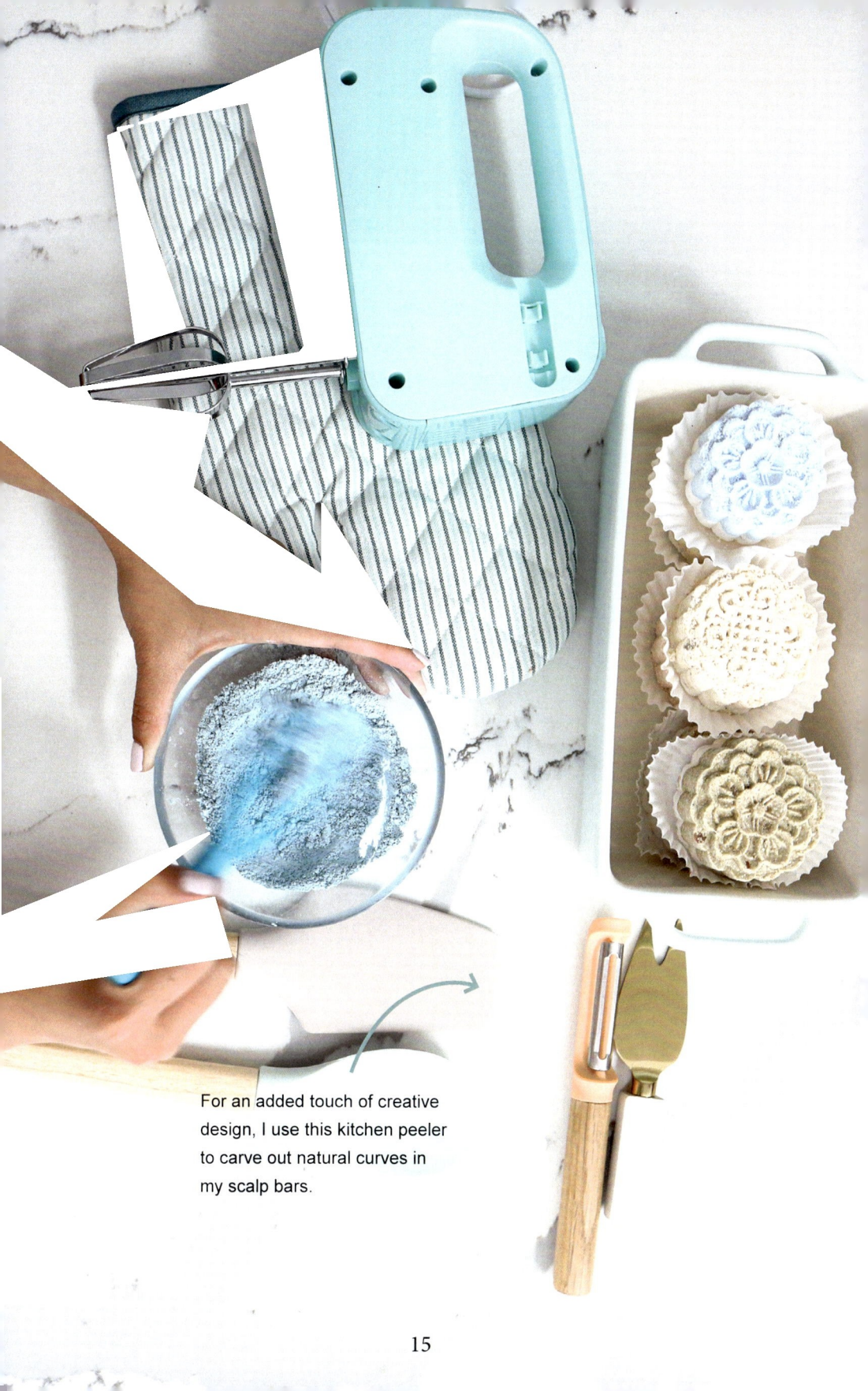

For an added touch of creative design, I use this kitchen peeler to carve out natural curves in my scalp bars.

How-to Guide

Pro-Tips + Tricks

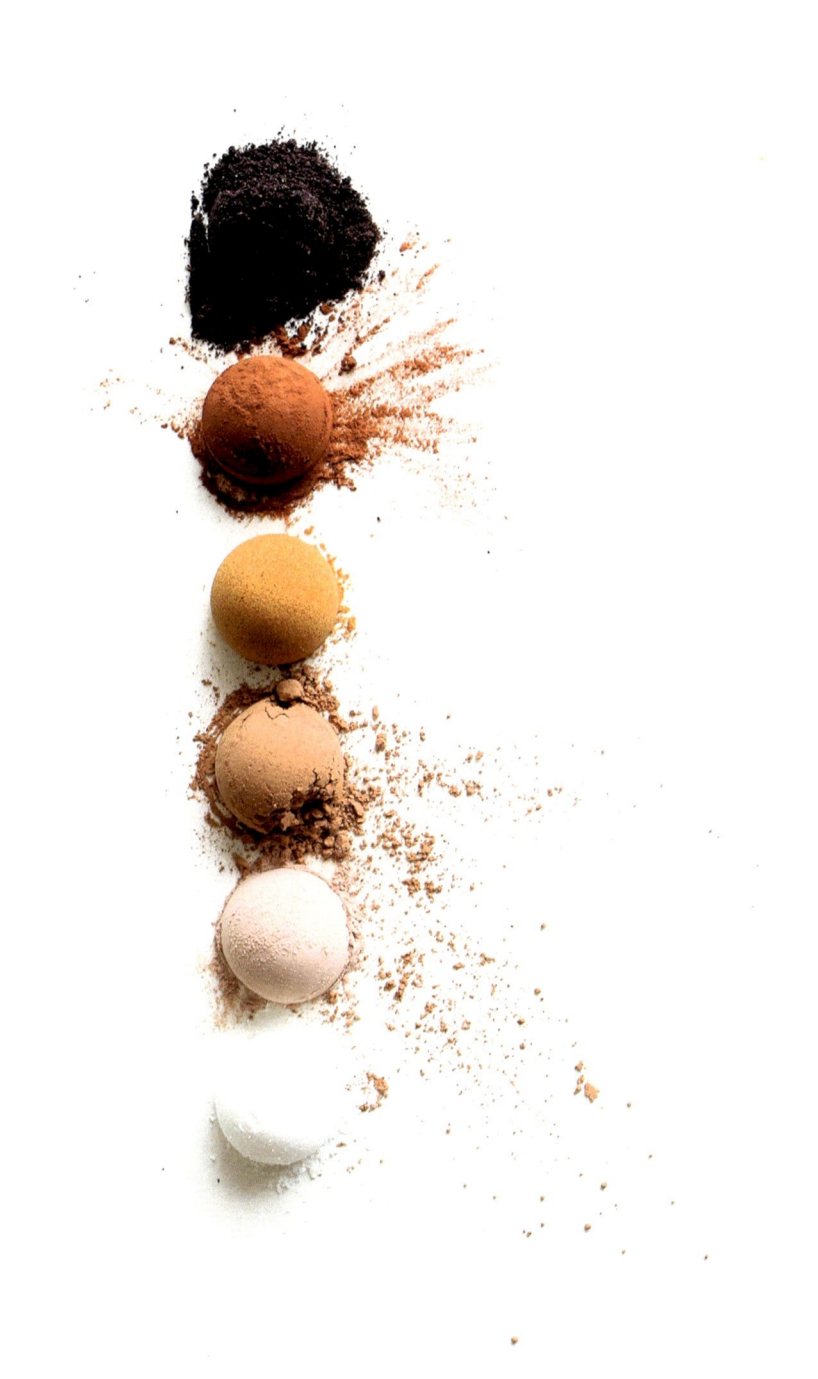

Guide to

Superfood Bronzers

How to Create Your Perfect Shade

Rose Blush

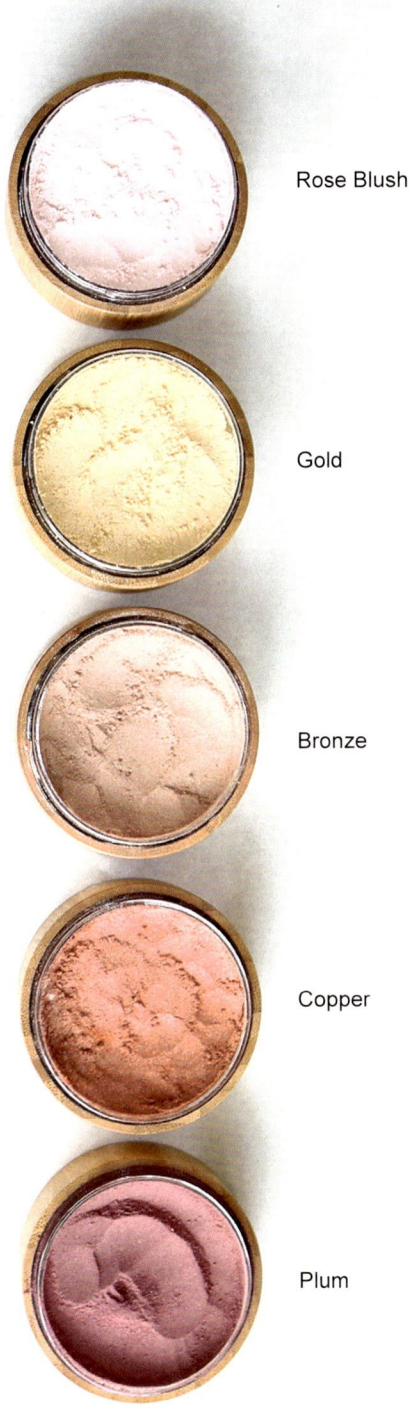

Gold

Bronze

Copper

Plum

Bronzers

Bronzers deliver a natural sun-kissed glow to the skin. A sweep of mineral superfood bronzer on the high points of your face creates subtle definition while also adding a beautiful, all over warmth. The beauty of working with raw superfoods, clays and micas is that you can **mix and match ingredients** to create the perfect shade, and feel good about what you're putting on your skin.

Step 1: Skin Tone and Micas
First, you'll want to choose a mineral mica powder based on your skin tone. If your goal is to create a bronzer, the general rule would be to choose a mica one or two shades darker than your natural skin tone. If your goal is to create a highlighter, select a mica powder that's one or two shades lighter than your skin tone.

Step 2: Skin Undertone and Superfood Powders
Superfood extract powders are not only packed with vitamins and antioxidants our skin craves, they're naturally colourful too! From warm pinks to cool blues, the trick is to find those that match your skin's undertone.

"So what's an undertone"? Undertones are the permanent, underlying color that your skin tone casts. There are three main buckets— warm, cool and neutral.

Warm undertones
If your skin has yellow, peach, or golden underlying colors you have warm undertones. Consider incorporating up to 4 superfoods with warm tones.
Tip: Where there is a toss up between superfood shades, look to their skin-boosting properties and antioxidants to determine which your skin needs more.

Cool undertones
If you have hints of pink or blue tones under your skin, consider ingredients with cooler tones. And don't forget, each superfood comes with it's own set of incredible properties including skin-loving vitamins and antioxidants.

Neutral undertones
If you see a mixture of both warm and cool tones in your skin, then your undertone is neutral.

Copper

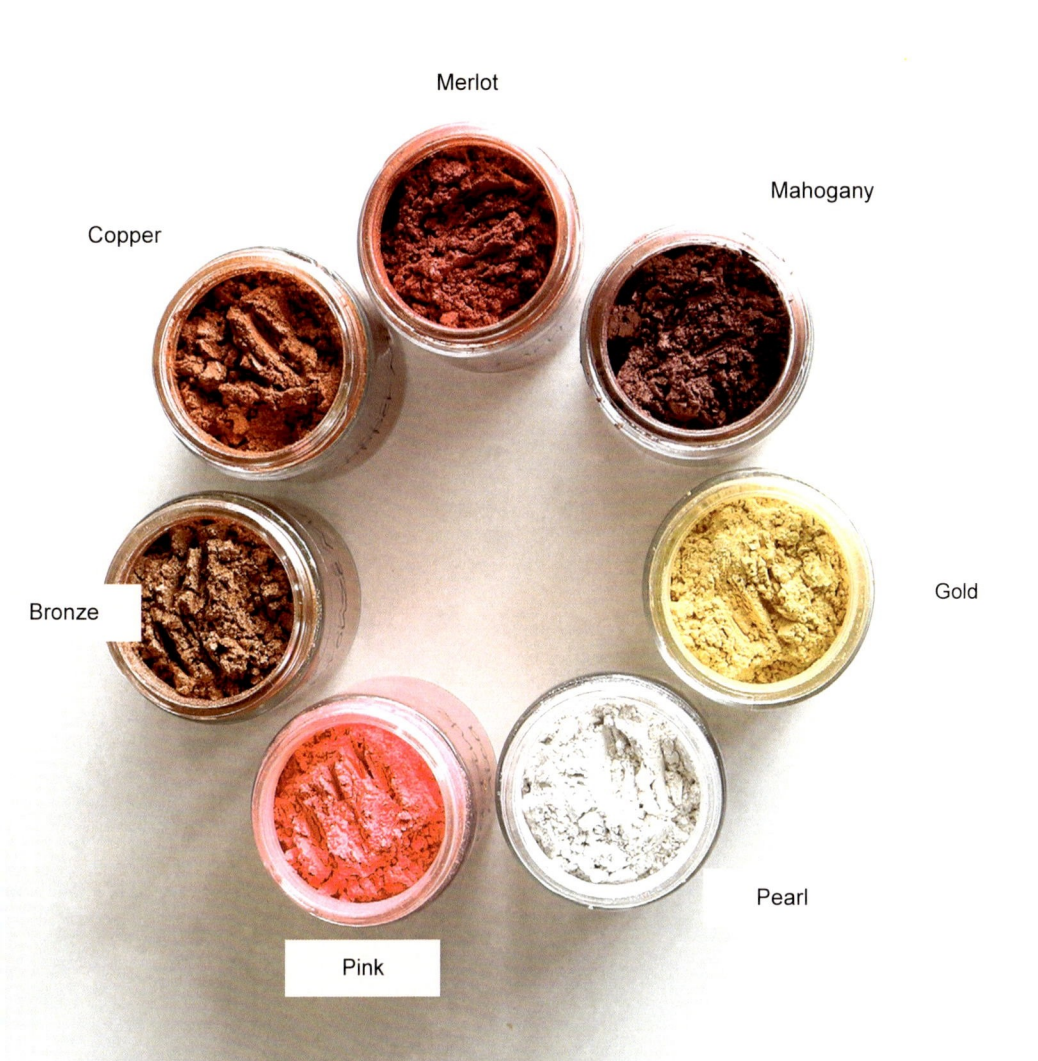

Merlot

Mahogany

Bronze

Gold

Pearl

Pink

Mineral Micas

Matcha

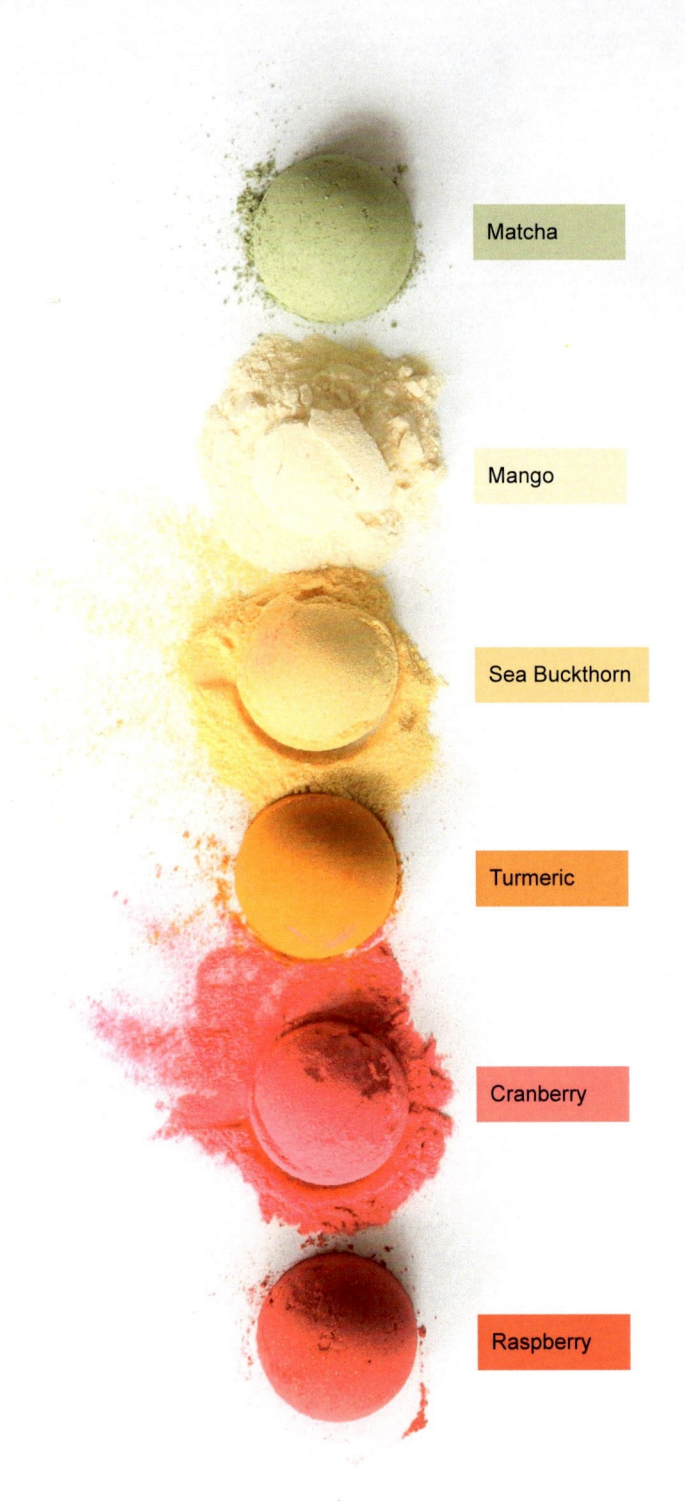

Mango

Sea Buckthorn

Turmeric

Cranberry

Raspberry

Warm Undertones

Green Spirulina

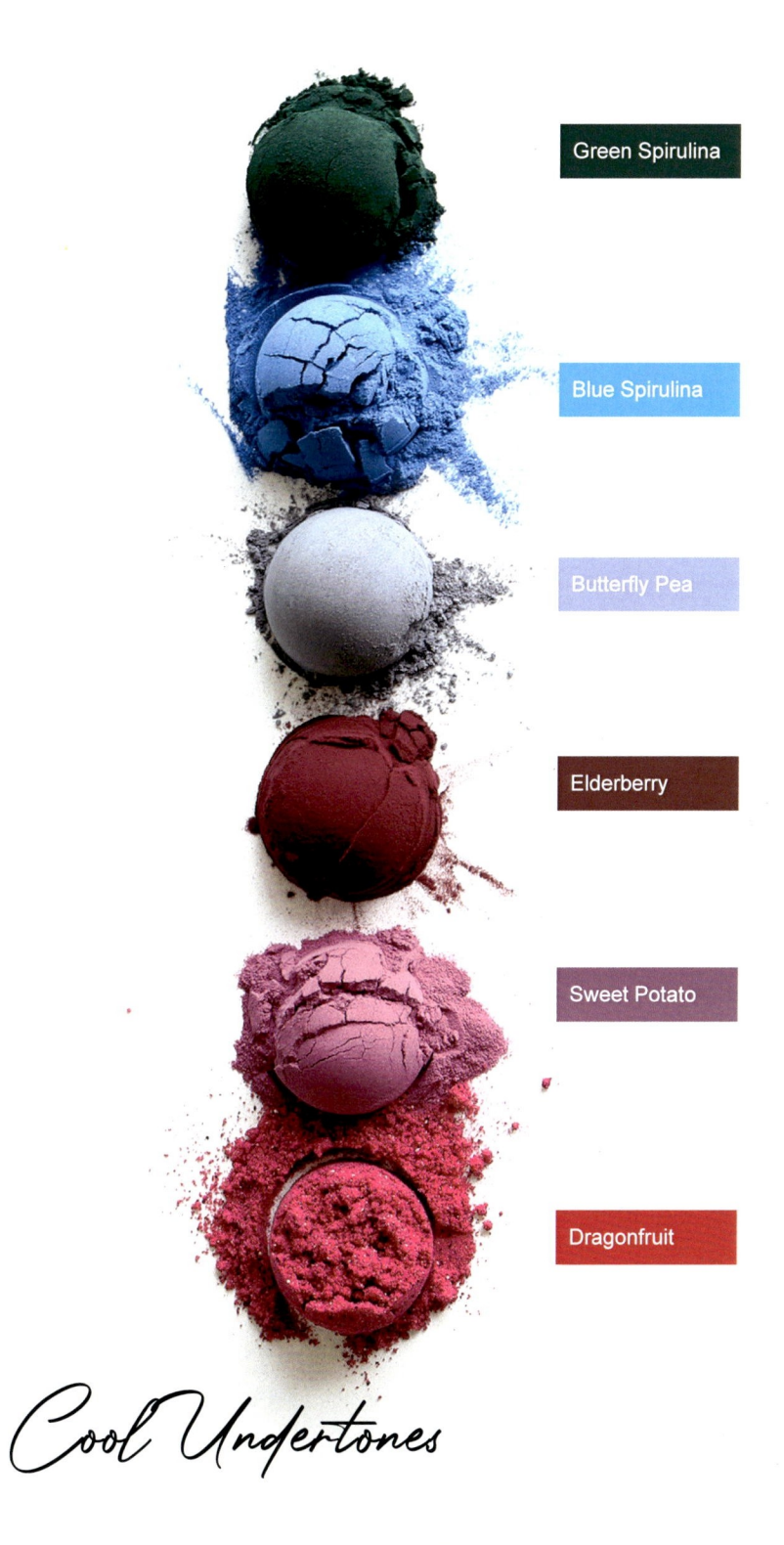

Blue Spirulina

Butterfly Pea

Elderberry

Sweet Potato

Dragonfruit

Cool Undertones

Apple Cider

Bamboo Leaf

Cocoa

Golden Berry

Grape Seed

Wolfberry

Neutral Undertones

STEP 3: Skin Undertones and Mineral Clays

The final customizable ingredient in your bronzer palette will be clay. Clays are chock-full of minerals (like magnesium) and detoxifying ingredients that can help with everything from acne to anti-aging. Clays come in different colours, for example green kaolin clay is green because it comes from clay that contains plant matter and has high levels of iron oxide. Find the clay shade that suits your skin's undertones.

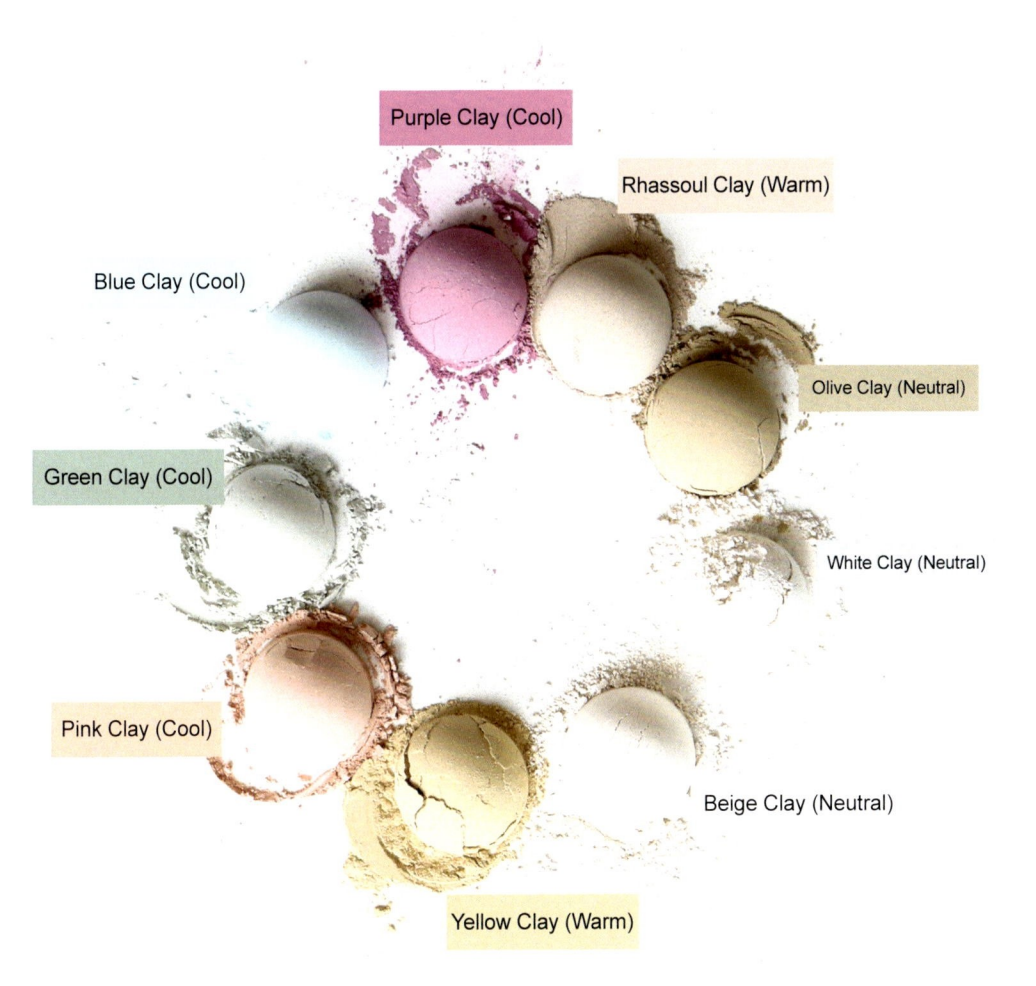

- Purple Clay (Cool)
- Rhassoul Clay (Warm)
- Blue Clay (Cool)
- Olive Clay (Neutral)
- Green Clay (Cool)
- White Clay (Neutral)
- Pink Clay (Cool)
- Beige Clay (Neutral)
- Yellow Clay (Warm)

Guide to

Streamlining your Diy Pantry like a Pro!

Minimize | Organize | Create

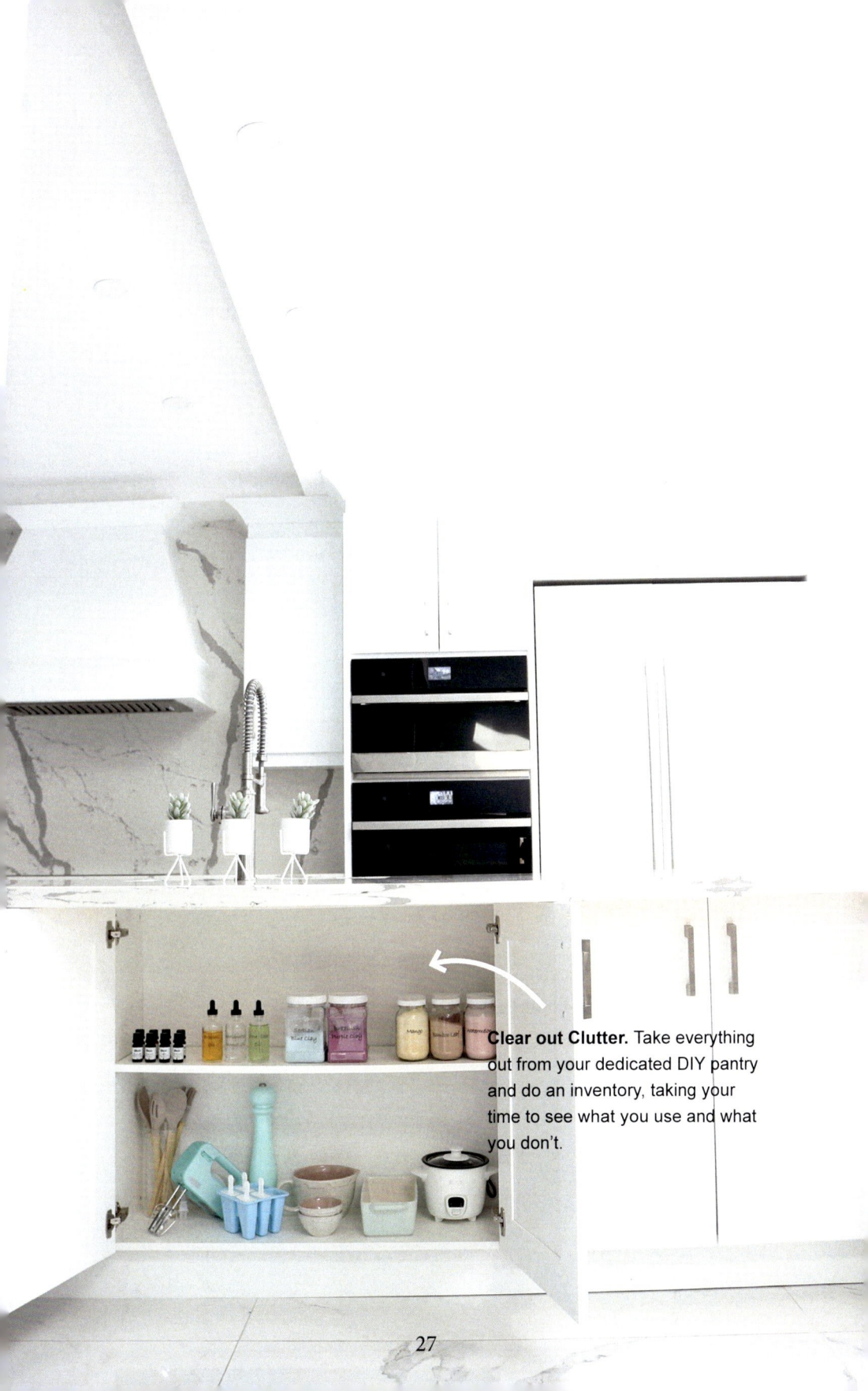

Clear out Clutter. Take everything out from your dedicated DIY pantry and do an inventory, taking your time to see what you use and what you don't.

Minimize and Organize your DIY Pantry

Whatever size pantry or space you have allotted for your ingredients is perfect. See it as a mindset shift that will allow you to pare down, streamline and let go of things you don't really need. There are certain ingredient categories that I cannot do without, and here they are.

1. Cold-Pressed Organic Carrier Oils
Carrier oils are a staple ingredient for so many luxurious recipes from cleansing oils to body oils to bath bombs. They are loaded with natural antioxidants from vitamins A to K, can be used straight up and are (for the most part) naturally unscented. I love to use apricot kernel as a simple cleansing oil and make-up remover because it's rich in vitamin K (for dark circles). Other carrier oils include argan, jojoba, carrot and grape seed.

2. Organic Essential Oils
Essential oils are loaded with antioxidants, beautiful aromas and mood-boosting benefits (we never use synthetic toxic fragrance oils). I like to keep a range of eo's and I group them by category: florals (Lavender and Rose), citrus (Orange and Lemon), earthy (Frankincense and Patchouli) and mint or herbs (Peppermint and Eucalyptus). *If you're new to essential oils and how they work, check out my sister's course on Udemy.com called Aromatherapy Foundations and Formulas, by Lana Marconi.*

3. Superfood Powders
Superfoods are the heart of most of my ingredients for very good reason— they're chock-full of skin-boosting antioxidants and vitamins, come in an array of beautiful colours and they have a great shelf life (as opposed to using fresh fruits and veggies which contain water). Some of my favourites include blue spirulina, cranberry and elderberry.

4. Raw Butters
Raw butters, like Shea and Cocoa are loaded with vitamins and essential fatty acids that our skin and hair crave. I'll use butters in everything from conditioners to eye creams to melting balms. There are so many beautiful and exotic type raw butters on the market like Murumuru, Cupuacu and Carrot. Did you know that Murumuru butter is considered nature's vegetable silicone, because it adds chemical-free shine and gloss to your hair products.

5. Mineral Clays
Clays are natural exfoliators, cleansers, detoxifiers and can even hydrate the skin (like Rhassoul clay). We use clays in our soaps, masks, bronzers and they come in an array of beautiful natural colours.

6. Melt and Pour Natural Soap Bases
Melt and pour is not just for kids. It's the perfect ingredient for creating luxurious all-natural cleansing bars, scalp bars, facial bars and more. Today, there are so many varieties of melt and pour soaps on the market that you can try— from Shea and Argan to Aloe and Honey.

7. Physical Raw Exfoliants
You probably already have and use superfood exfoliants in your kitchen. Look for things like coffee grinds, chia seeds and flax seeds. These grit-based physical exfoliators add an extra dose of exfoliation strength where needed.

8. Mineral Salts
Sugar is out, salt is in! Mineral salts like Dead Sea Salt and Pink Himalayan are super rich in minerals our body needs. In fact, Pink Himalayan has over 84 trace minerals and Dead Sea has around 21 (like magnesium, potassium). I use salts in plenty of my recipes, from bath soaks and body scrubs to milk bath fizzes and bath bombs.

9. Baking Staples
Arrowroot powder, coconut powder, citric acid powder and sodium bicarbonate (baking powder) are simple yet effective ingredients. I'll use arrowroot in my bronzing powders, coconut powder in masks and citric acid powder in bath bombs. Check your kitchen pantry as you may already have these staple ingredients.

10. Mineral Earth Micas
Mica powder creates a natural shimmery finish, is brightening and illuminating. Colours vary between the different micas, from silver and pink to yellow, purple and brown tones. Finding a natural and sustainable source (fair trade) for your mica (and all ingredients for that matter) is key. Mica can be used in our make-up recipes including bronzing powders and lip luminizers.

11. Waxes
Waxes are a very useful ingredient that can help thicken a product, add gloss and provide stability— think about lip balms and deodorants. Beeswax is a very common wax but there are vegan wax options too, like Candelilla and Carnauba. The difference lies in their melting point. If you create water and oil recipes, you will require a self-emulsifying wax to bind the water and oil ingredients.

12. Natural Preservative
When creating water and oil recipes you will need a natural preservative to protect your water-based product from bacteria, yeast and mold growth. We love working with Leucidal Liquid Complete as our natural preservative.

13. Natural Cream Bases
For those who don't want to bother with water, oil and preservatives (and testing) do not fret— you have options! Try ready-made natural butter bases. They come professionally mixed with clean ingredients and preservatives. Simply mix in your additives and ta-da!

DECANT

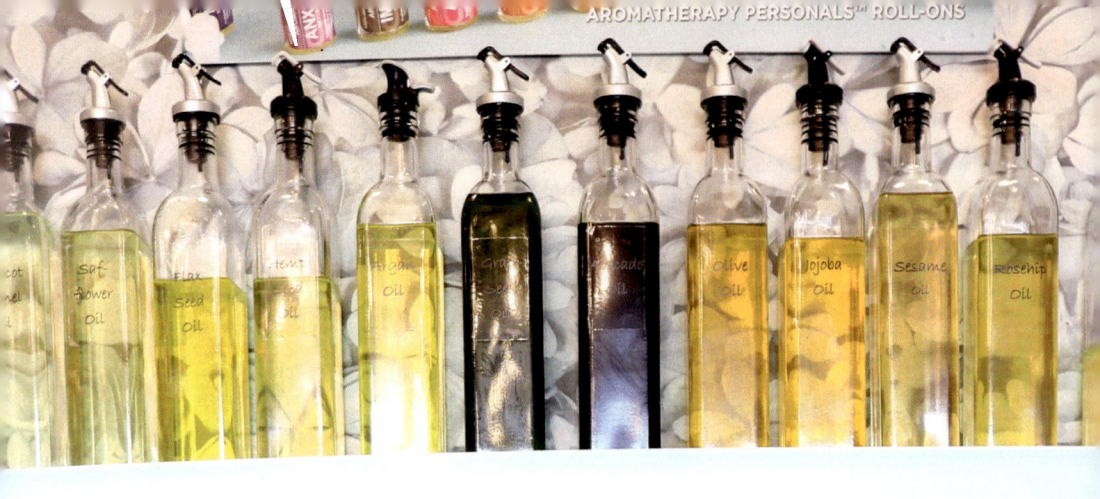

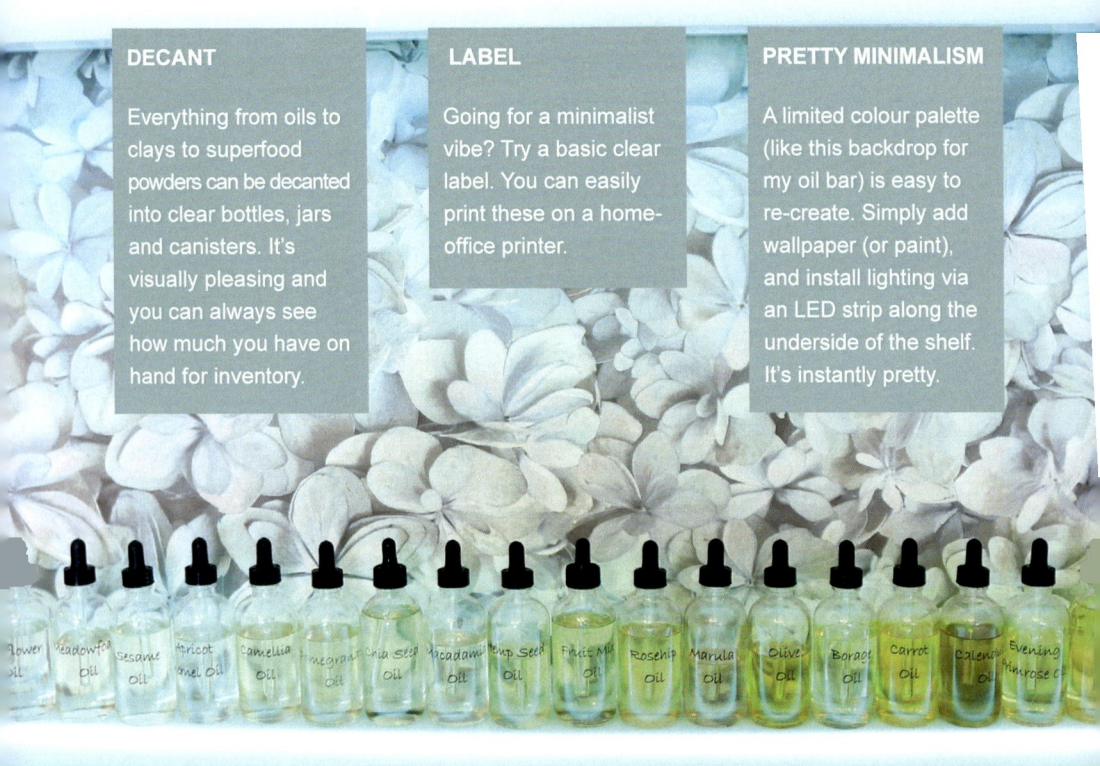

Everything from oils to clays to superfood powders can be decanted into clear bottles, jars and canisters. It's visually pleasing and you can always see how much you have on hand for inventory.

LABEL

Going for a minimalist vibe? Try a basic clear label. You can easily print these on a home-office printer.

PRETTY MINIMALISM

A limited colour palette (like this backdrop for my oil bar) is easy to re-create. Simply add wallpaper (or paint), and install lighting via an LED strip along the underside of the shelf. It's instantly pretty.

Decluttering is the goal. It saves time, improves productivity and the creative process. You can apply these same simple organizing tips that I use in my store, to set the tone for your DIY kitchen pantry.

A Pro-Streamlined Space

STREAMLINED STORAGE TIPS: THE TOOLS
The storage principles for your DIY tools are the same whether it's for your home or business.

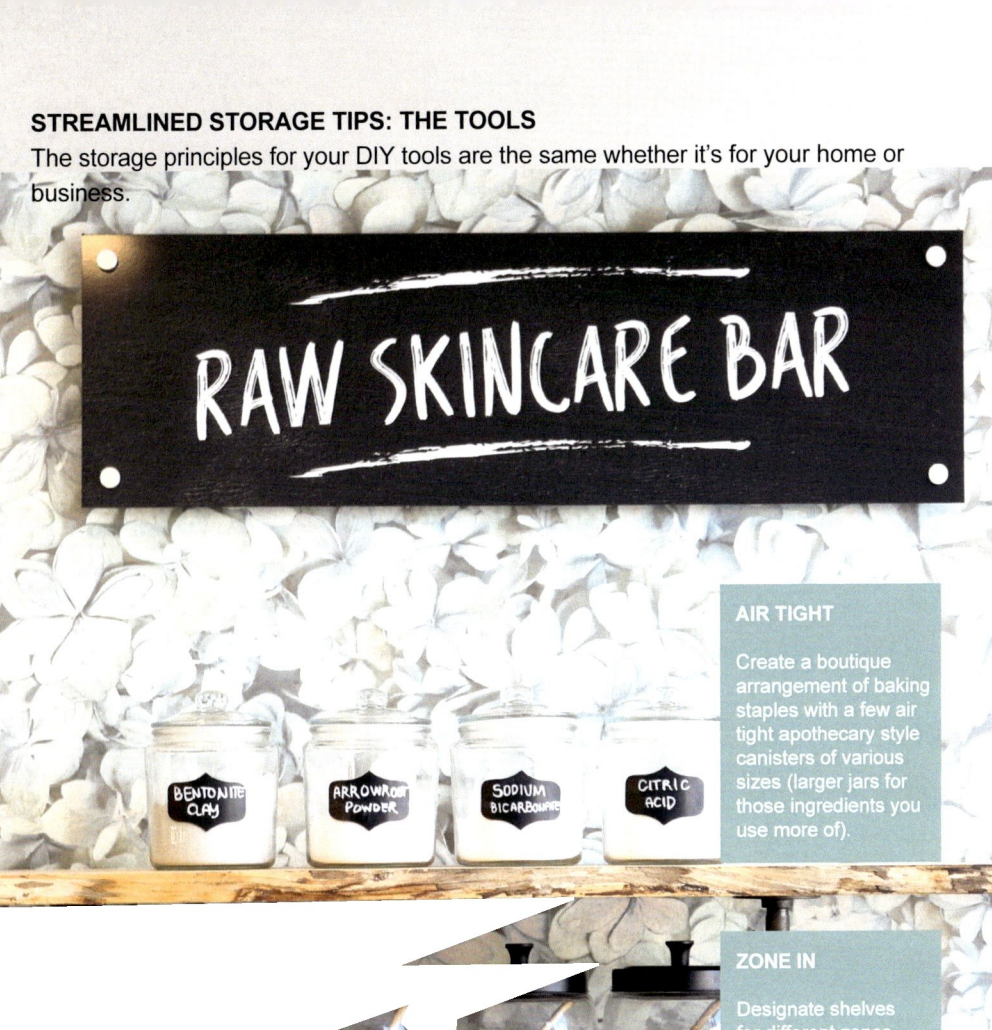

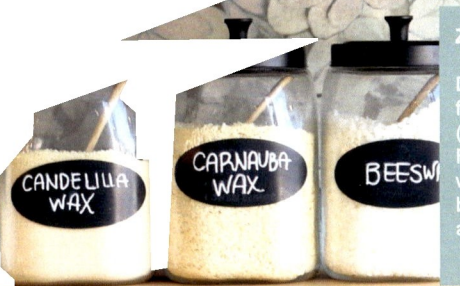

RAW SKINCARE BAR

AIR TIGHT
Create a boutique arrangement of baking staples with a few air tight apothecary style canisters of various sizes (larger jars for those ingredients you use more of).

ZONE IN
Designate shelves for different zones (Ingredient categories). For example, keep waxes with waxes, butters with butters and so forth.

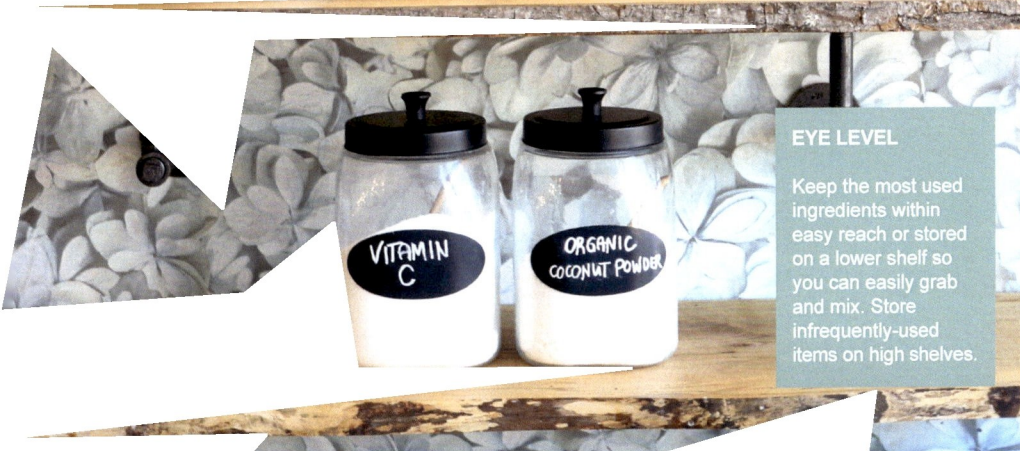

EYE LEVEL
Keep the most used ingredients within easy reach or stored on a lower shelf so you can easily grab and mix. Store infrequently-used items on high shelves.

31

Our

Superfood Colour Guide

Set the tone for your product colour scheme

COLOUR-CODING

Superfood powders come in so many beautiful natural colours. Decant into clear jars and then group your superfood powders by colour (check the pantone wheel). This will help you visualize the colours and hues that you want for your product creations.

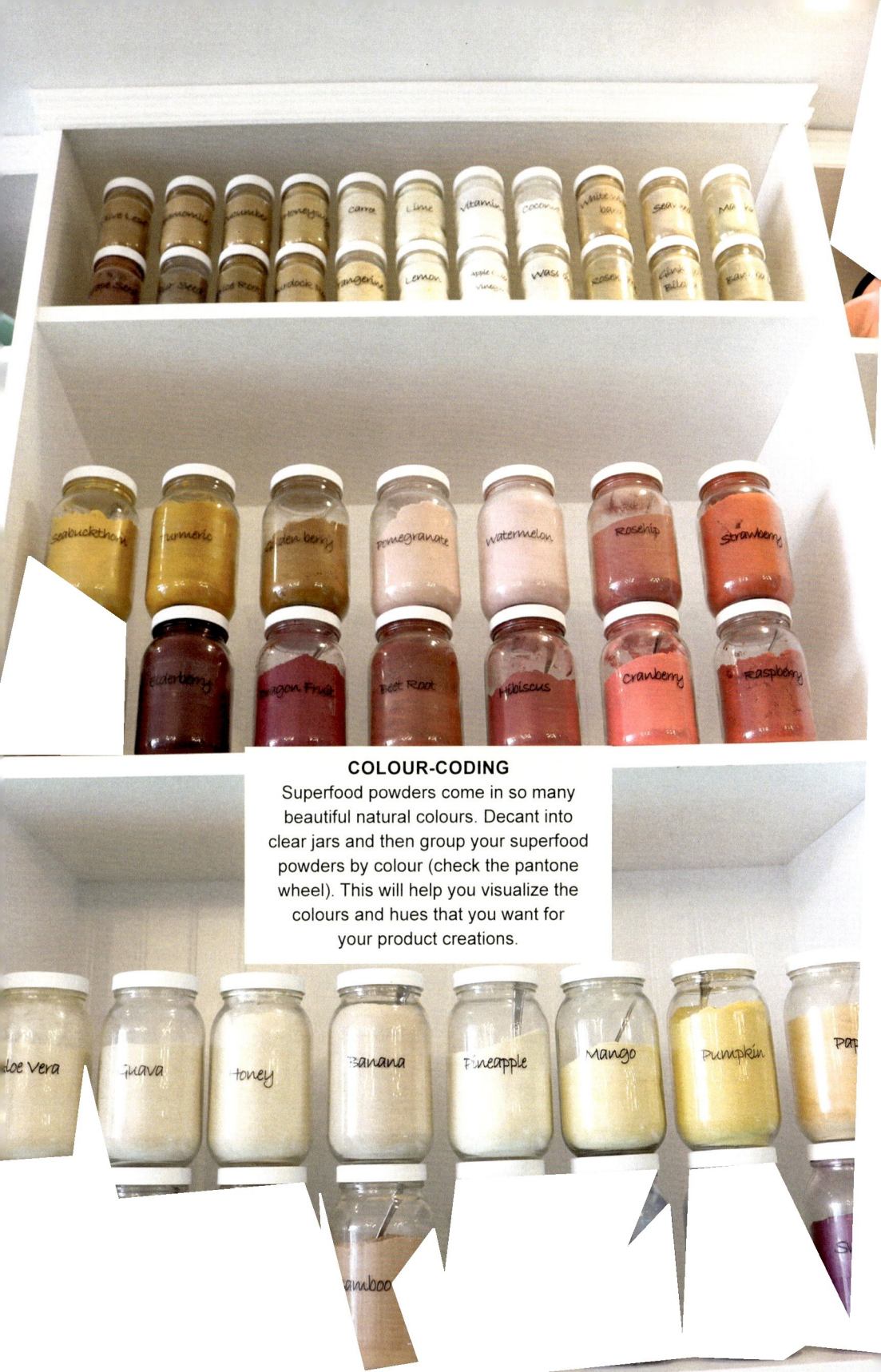

DIY Raspberry Body Butter Cream

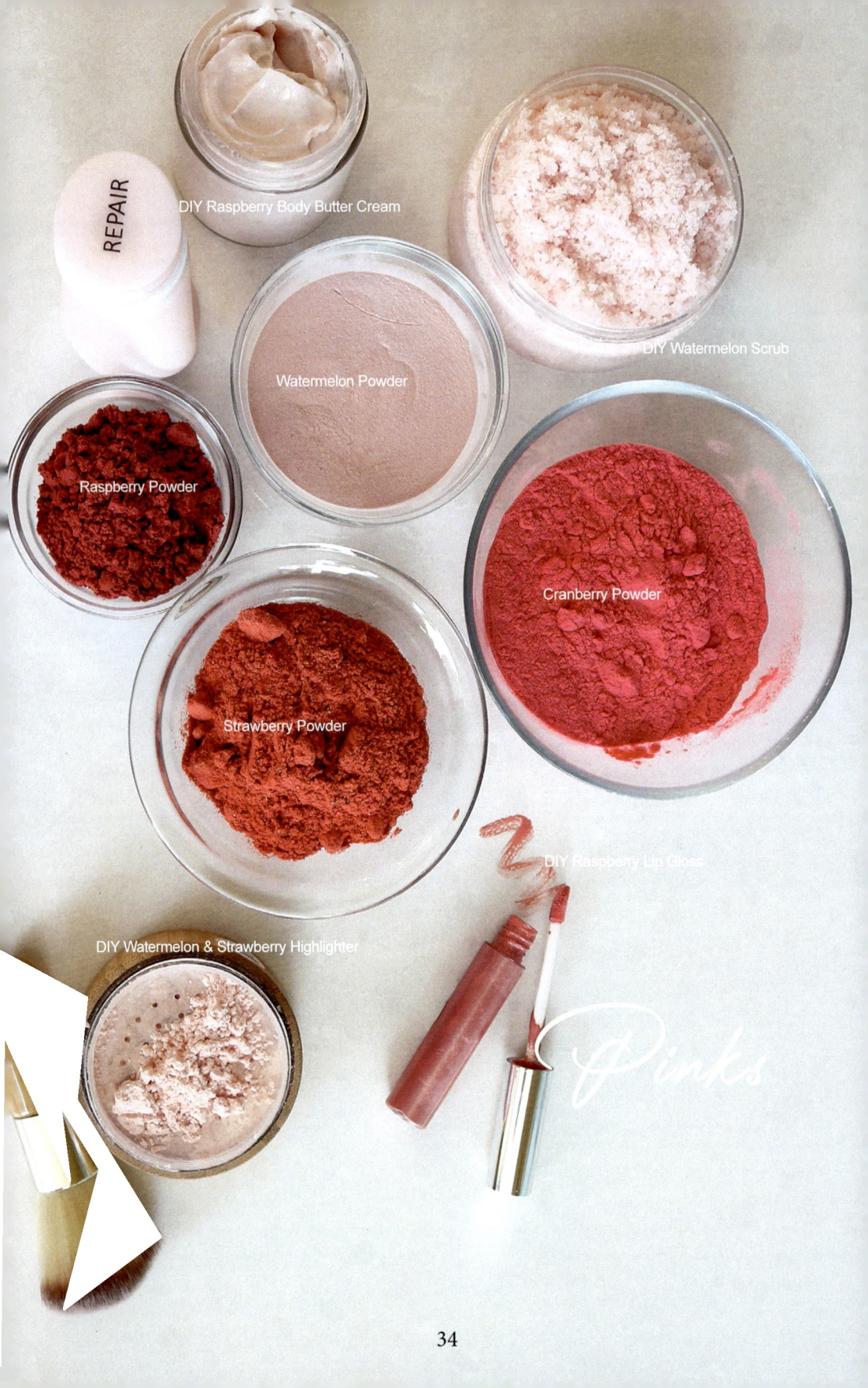

DIY Watermelon Scrub

Watermelon Powder

Raspberry Powder

Cranberry Powder

Strawberry Powder

DIY Raspberry Lip Gloss

DIY Watermelon & Strawberry Highlighter

Pinks

DIY Blueberry Bronzer

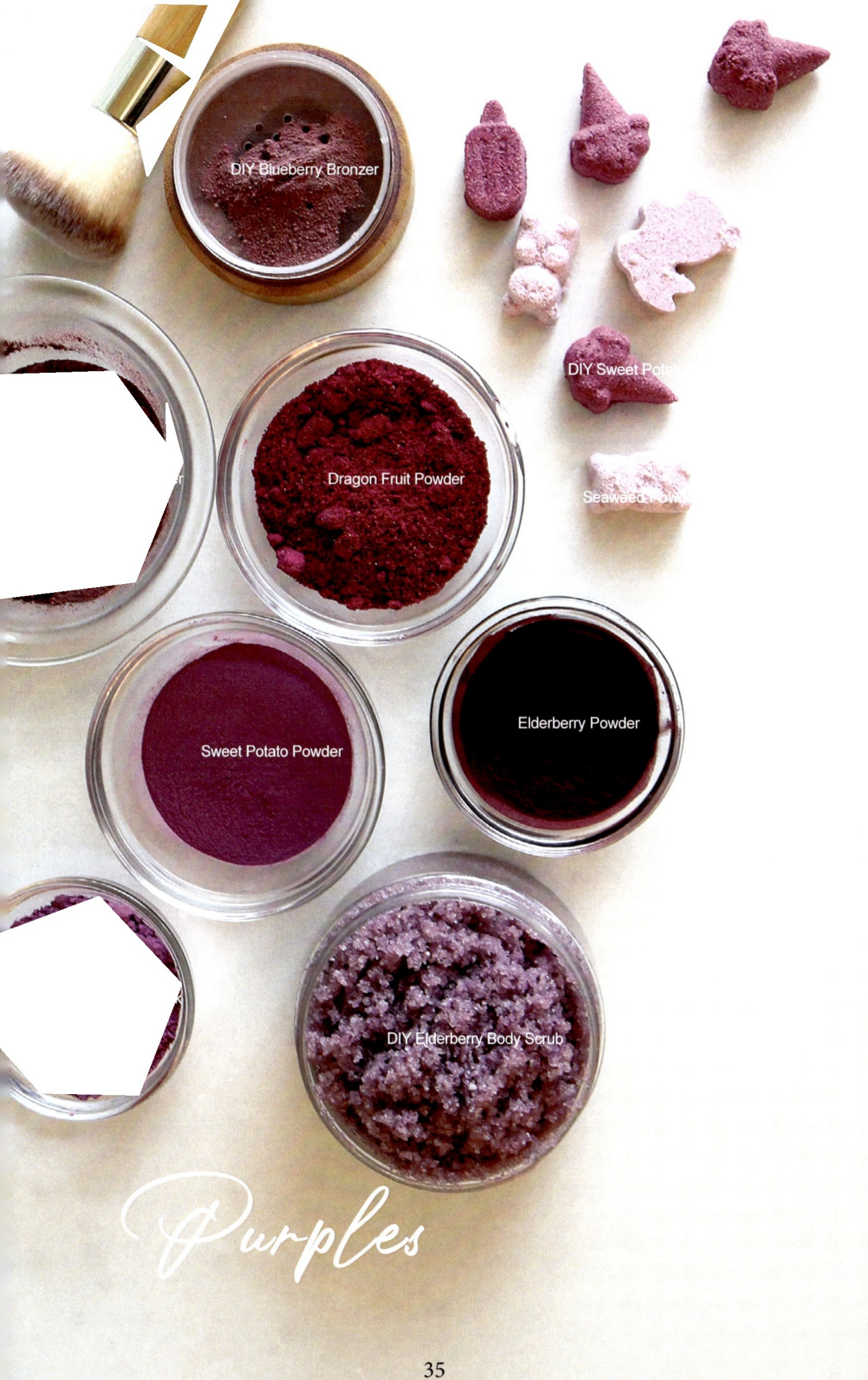

DIY Sweet Potato

Dragon Fruit Powder

Seaweed Powder

Elderberry Powder

Sweet Potato Powder

DIY Elderberry Body Scrub

Purples

DIY Banaba Scalp Bar

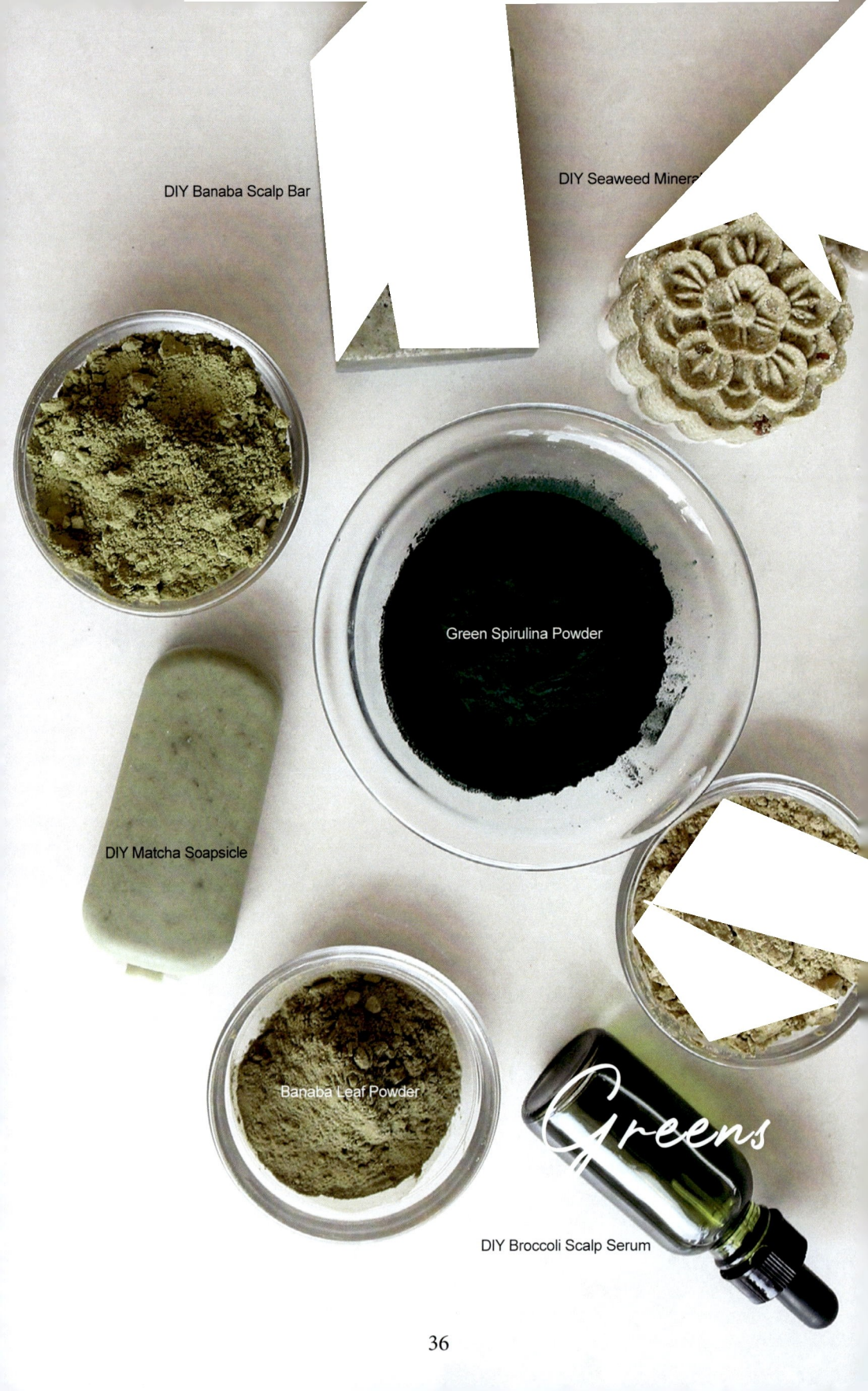

DIY Seaweed Mineral

Green Spirulina Powder

DIY Matcha Soapsicle

Banaba Leaf Powder

DIY Broccoli Scalp Serum

Greens

DIY Butterfly Pea Soapsicle

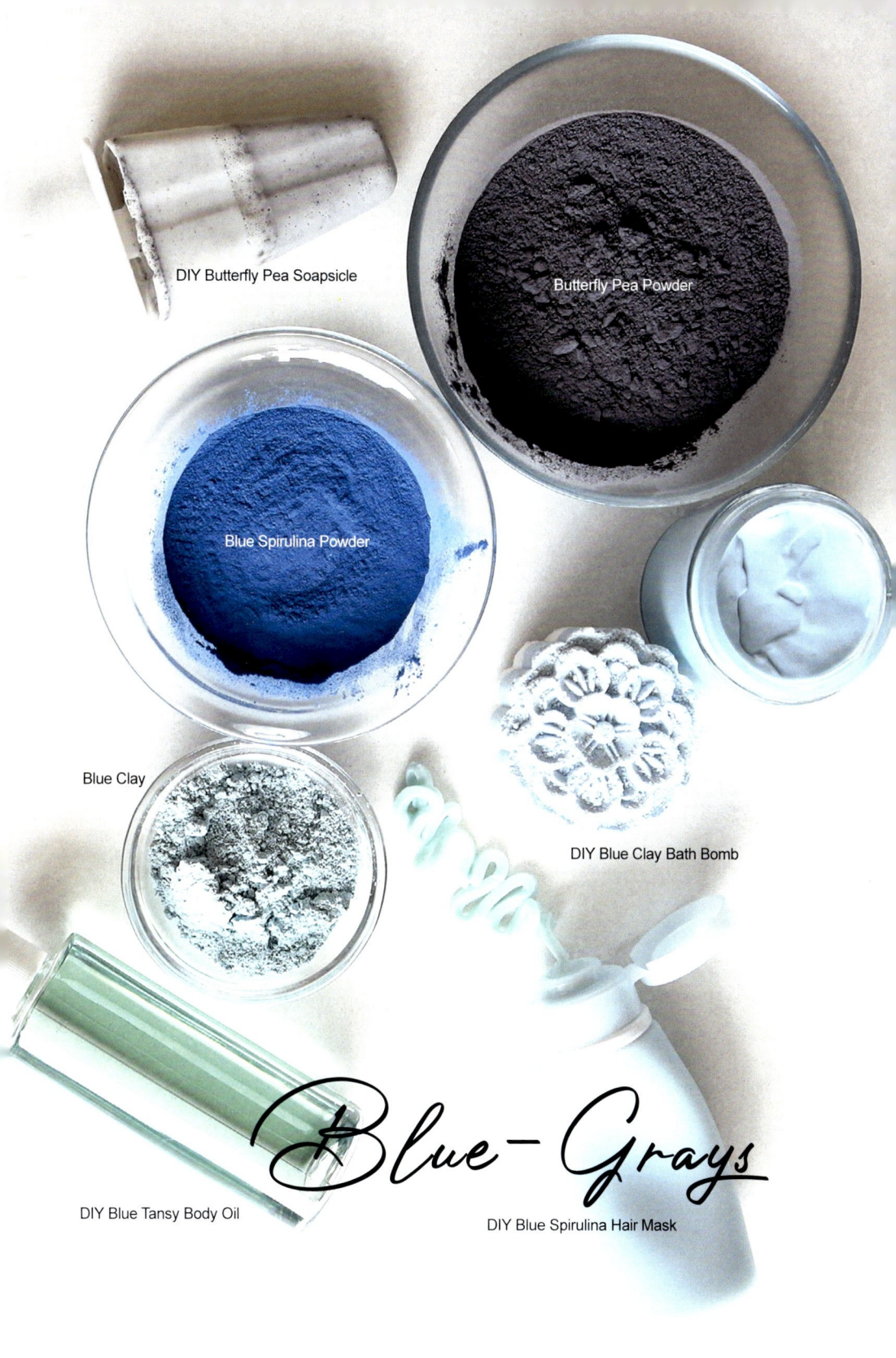

Butterfly Pea Powder

Blue Spirulina Powder

Blue Clay

DIY Blue Clay Bath Bomb

Blue-Grays

DIY Blue Tansy Body Oil

DIY Blue Spirulina Hair Mask

DIY Papaya Soapsicle

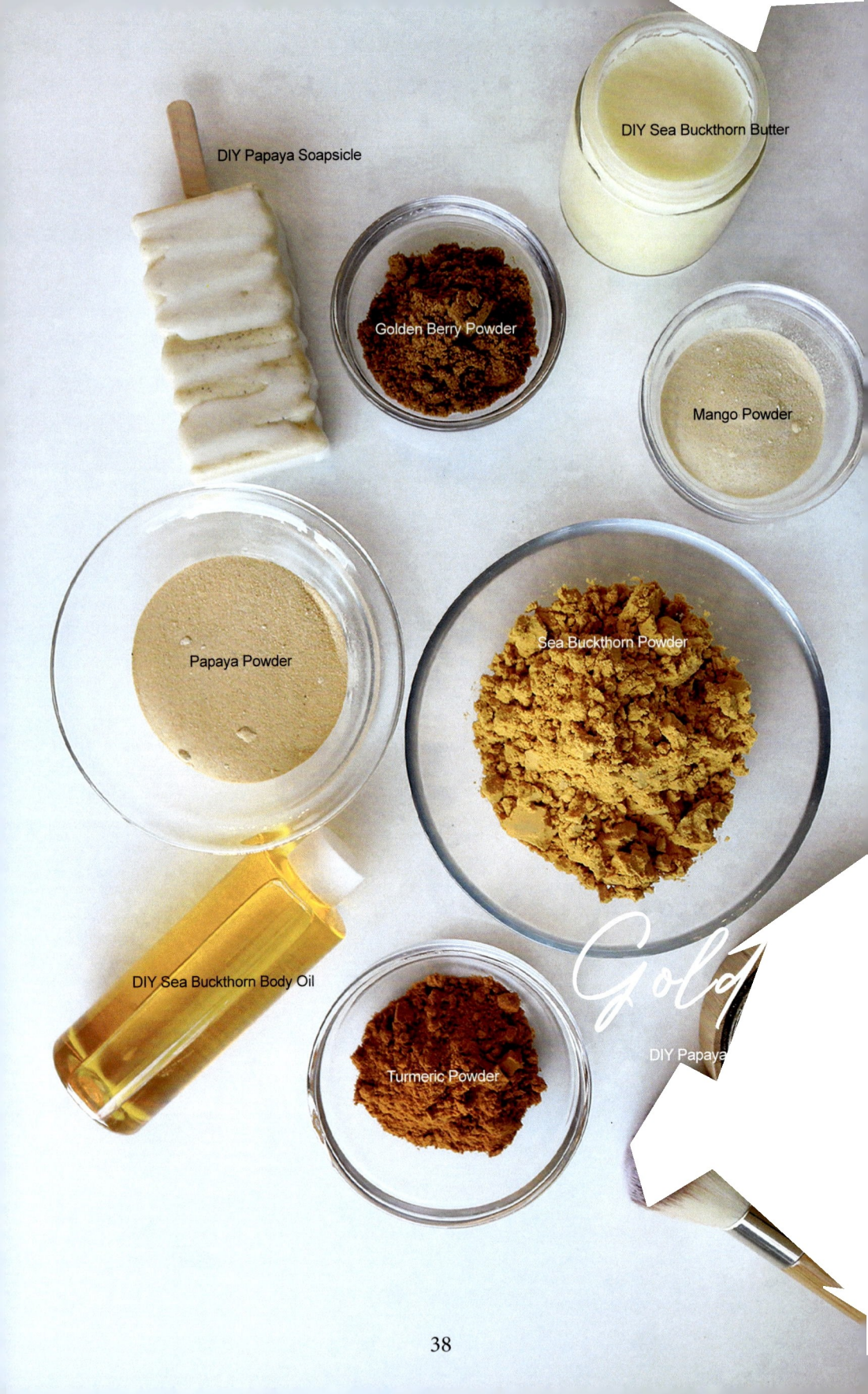

DIY Sea Buckthorn Butter

Golden Berry Powder

Mango Powder

Papaya Powder

Sea Buckthorn Powder

DIY Sea Buckthorn Body Oil

Turmeric Powder

Gold

DIY Papaya

Bamboo Charcoal Powder

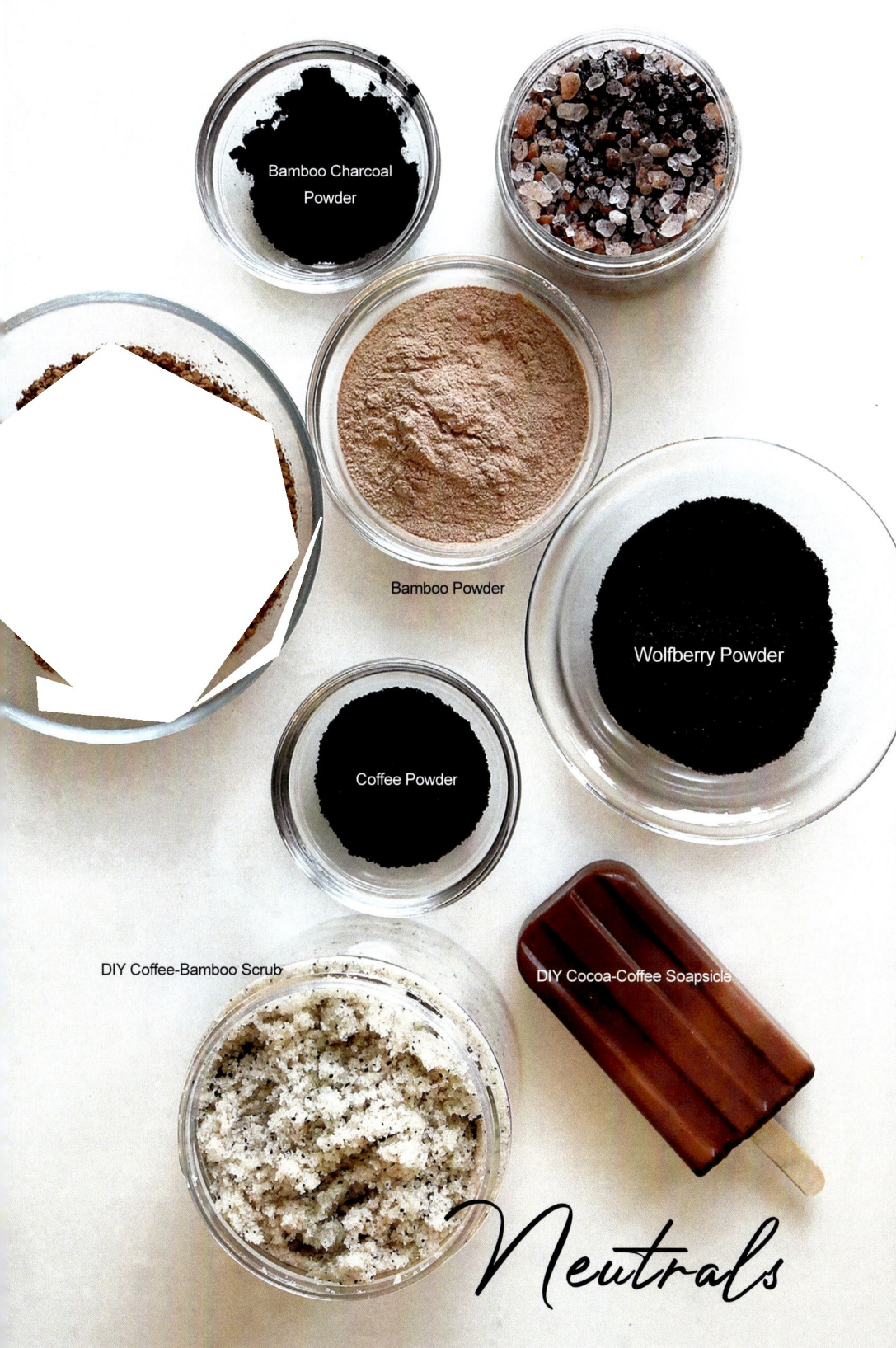

Bamboo Powder

Wolfberry Powder

Coffee Powder

DIY Coffee-Bamboo Scrub

DIY Cocoa-Coffee Soapsicle

Neutrals

Off-Whites

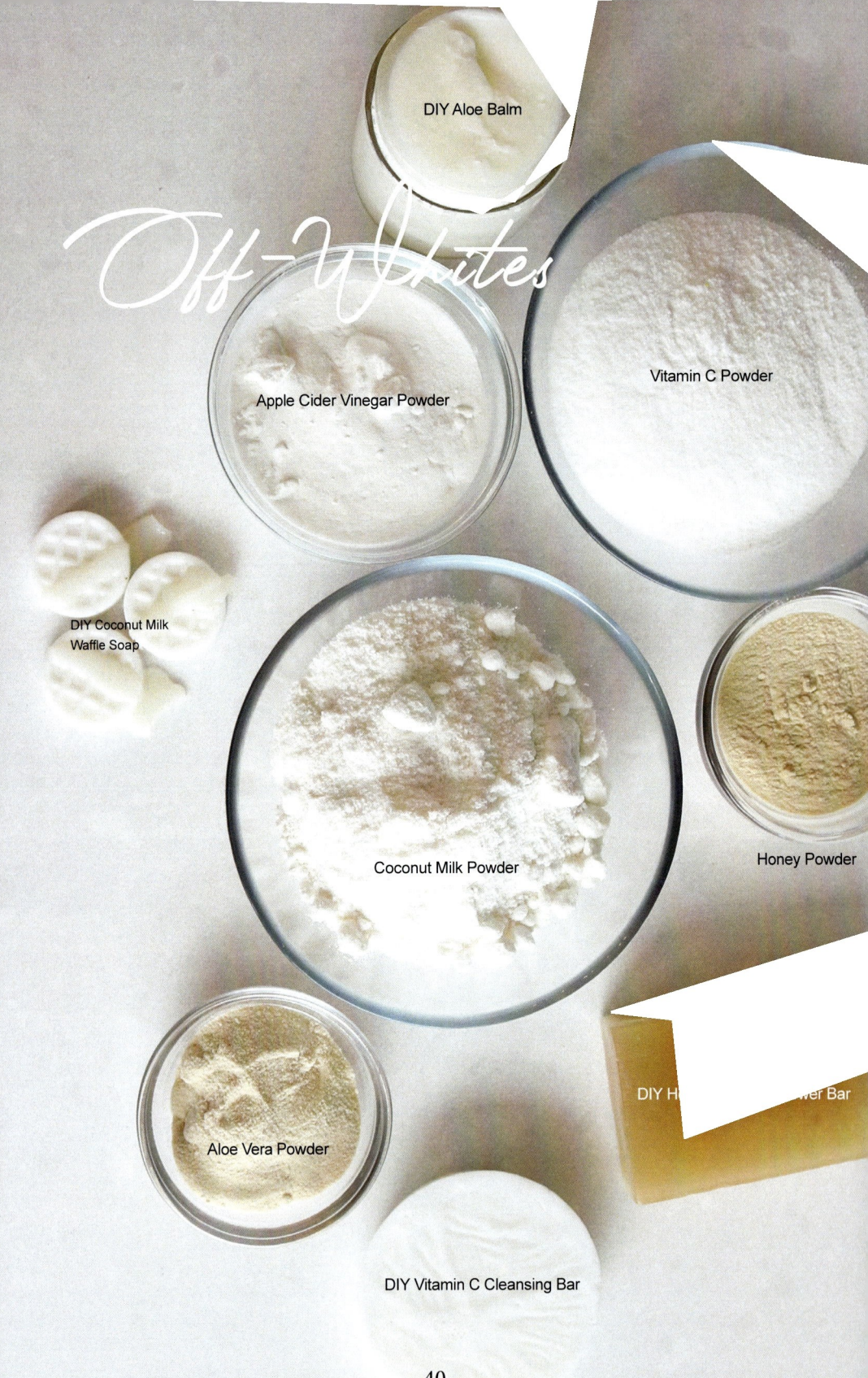

- DIY Aloe Balm
- Apple Cider Vinegar Powder
- Vitamin C Powder
- DIY Coconut Milk Waffle Soap
- Coconut Milk Powder
- Honey Powder
- Aloe Vera Powder
- DIY Honey Shower Bar
- DIY Vitamin C Cleansing Bar

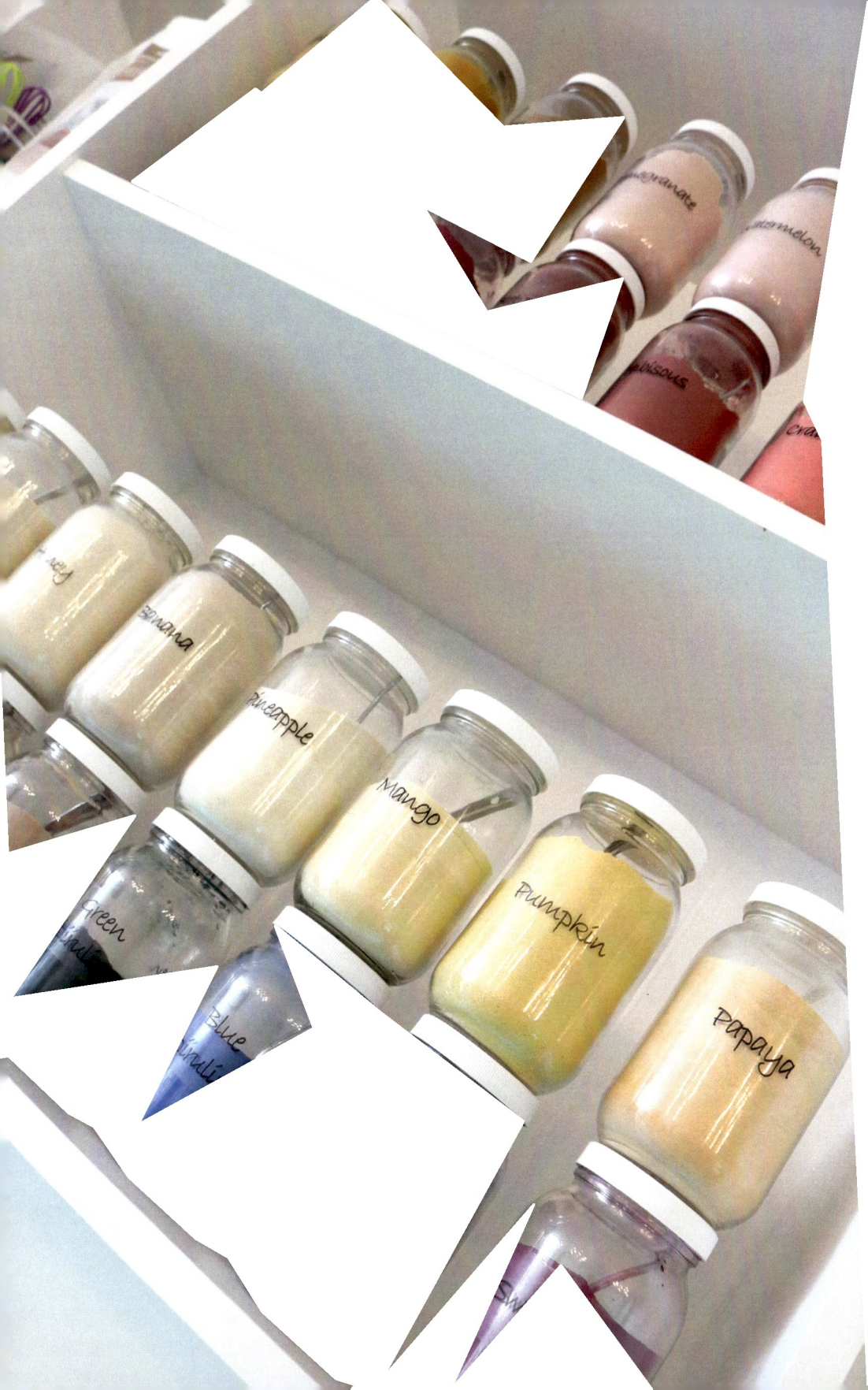

banana
Pineapple
Mango
Pumpkin
Papaya
Green
Blue
Pomegranate
watermelon
hibiscus

Guide to
Natural Source Alpha Hydroxy Acids + Vitamins

Natural Source AHA for Skincare

Alpha Hydroxy Acids (AHAs and BHAs) are super hero ingredients found in many anti-acne and anti-aging skincare products and are used to exfoliate your skin. They're known for smoothening, brightening and plumping the skin.

AHAs are the most common acids like glycolic acid, citric acid and lactic acid. These acids are typically used to exfoliate the outer layer of the skin, leaving the skin brighter, evening out skin tone and texture (ie hyperpigmentation) and stimulating collagen production (increasing plumpness and tightening of the skin). Beta-Hydroxy Acids (BHA) like salicylic acid are an acne-fighting ingredient.

Let's break it down:

Citric Acids. Citric acids come from fruit acids. These larger compounds work on the uppermost layer of the skin, and are often combined with glycolic or lactic acids to help boost their effectiveness. Plant source ingredients include citric fruits such as lemon powder and lemon essential oil, lime powder and lime essential oils, tangerine superfood powder, grapefruit essential oil and others.

Glycolic acid. Glycolic acid is derived from sugar cane. It regenerates collagen, evens out the skin tone and can help lessen the appearance of superficial scars and hyperpigmentation. It can be found in many common fruits and vegetables like beets, pineapples, papaya, and all kinds of citrus fruits.

Lactic acid. Lactic acid is one of the more gentle hydroxy acids that actually draws moisture to the skin (think milk baths). It is naturally found in milk, fruit, veggies and other plants. Lactic acid can help brighten the skin and improve the look of fine lines and wrinkles, because it stimulates collagen production. Powdered coconut milk is a natural source of lactic acid and when applied to the skin it is very effective in smoothing, toning and tightening the skin. The lactic acid found in apple cider vinegar powder can help soften and exfoliate skin, reduce red spots, and balance the pH of your skin.

Salicylic Acid. Salicylic acid is one of the best options for acne-prone skin. It penetrates and dissolves the oil that clogs pores while also exfoliating away dead skin cells. Willow bark powder contains salicin, which is where salicylic acid comes from. Turmeric also serves as a natural source of salicylic acid, a well-known ingredient in acne-prone treatments, which can be highly beneficial in regulating excessive sebum secretion. Other ingredients include broccoli oil, sweet potato extract, beet root extract and pumpkin extract.

CITRIC ACID

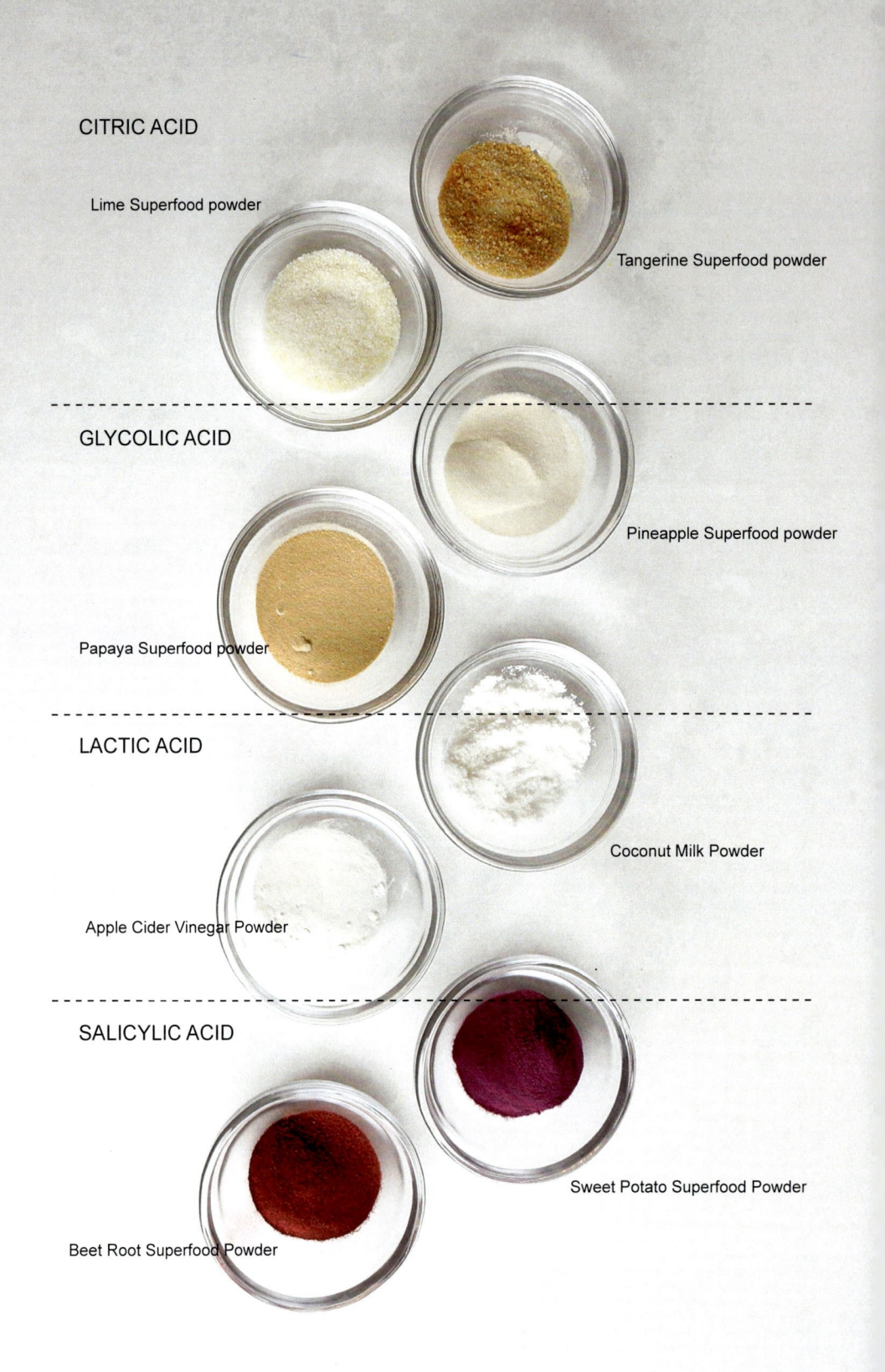

Lime Superfood powder

Tangerine Superfood powder

GLYCOLIC ACID

Pineapple Superfood powder

Papaya Superfood powder

LACTIC ACID

Coconut Milk Powder

Apple Cider Vinegar Powder

SALICYLIC ACID

Sweet Potato Superfood Powder

Beet Root Superfood Powder

Add a bit of grit to your products with a physical exfoliant. One of the mildest exfoliants we use is jojoba beads; and one of the strongest exfoliants is apricot shells. Choose the right exfoliant to suit your product type and take into consideration whether the product will be used on the face or body.

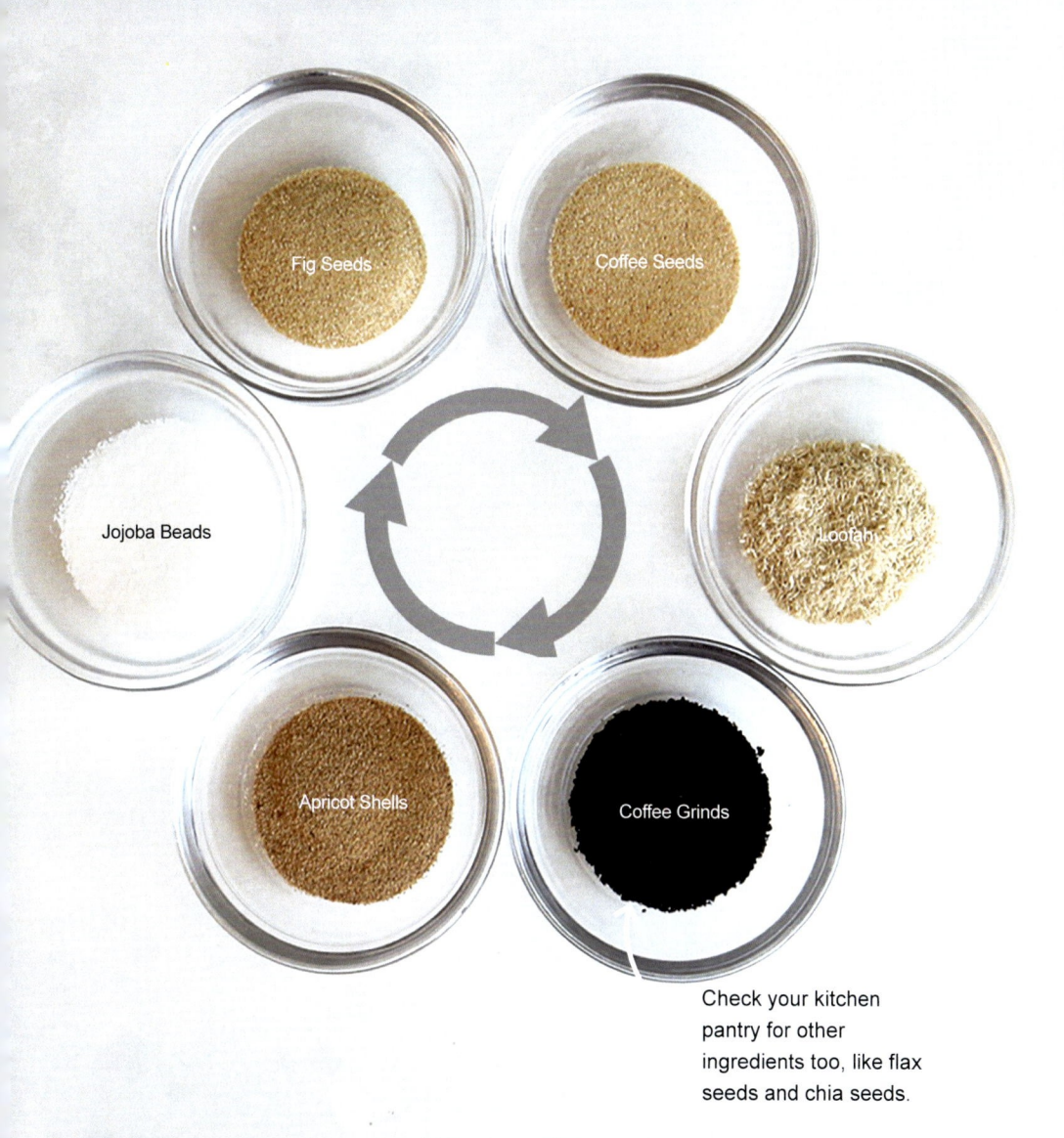

Fig Seeds

Coffee Seeds

Jojoba Beads

Loofah

Apricot Shells

Coffee Grinds

Check your kitchen pantry for other ingredients too, like flax seeds and chia seeds.

Physical Exfoliators

45

Vitamin A

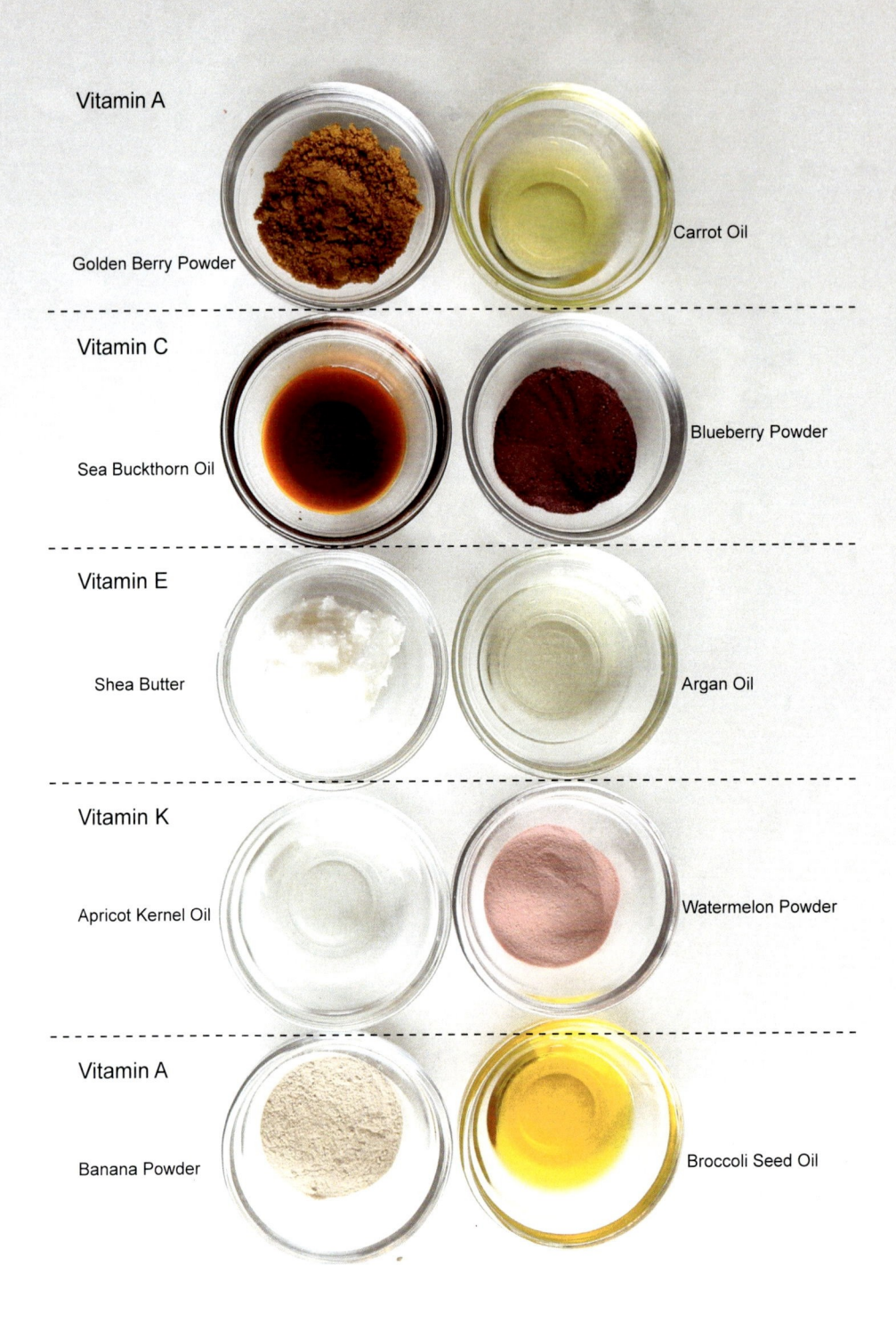

Golden Berry Powder

Carrot Oil

Vitamin C

Sea Buckthorn Oil

Blueberry Powder

Vitamin E

Shea Butter

Argan Oil

Vitamin K

Apricot Kernel Oil

Watermelon Powder

Vitamin A

Banana Powder

Broccoli Seed Oil

Natural Source Vitamins: Oils I Powders I Butters

Vitamin A– Vitamin A is very effective at reducing fine lines and wrinkles by increasing the production of collagen. It can also help with scarring, acne, hyperpigmentation, skin texture and your skin's hydration levels. Natural vitamin A can be found in many plant-based ingredients including rosehip oil, raspberry oil, murumuru butter, sea buckthorn oil, golden berry powder, sweet potato powder and carrot oil.

Vitamin C– Vitamin C is touted as one of the best ultra-protective, anti-aging ingredients on the market. As well as being a reliable multi-tasker, it's also the key to maintaining a smooth, even, and glowing complexion. From uneven skin tone and fine lines to acne scars and general dullness, there is a good chance that vitamin C can help you out. Some examples include aloe vera powder, sea buckthorn powder, tangerine powder, lemon oil, pineapple powder, pomegranate oil and blueberry powder.

Vitamin E– Vitamin E helps skin stay moisturized and supple. It can help fight inflammation and heal dry patchy skin. It also strengthens the skin barrier. Natural plant-source ingredients with vitamin E are plentiful, like shea butter, cocoa butter, argan oil, hemp seed oil, safflower oil, avocado oil and jojoba oil.

Another type of vitamin E you will see in my recipes is vitamin E (MT-50 otherwise known as Tocopherol). This ingredient is a natural antioxidant with a full spectrum of tocopherols which will help extend the shelf-life of oils. This is an optional ingredient and good to include in some retail products.

Vitamin K– Superfruits can work wonders on dark circles. As we age, capillaries under the eye can become weak and break easily, causing it to darken under the skin. Ingredients packed with vitamin K can help shrink capillaries and reduce the visibility of dark circles, spider veins, redness and even age spots. Oils that are rich in vitamin K include broccoli oil, olive oil, apricot kernel oil and blueberry oil. Superfood powders include watermelon, cucumber, blueberry, golden berry and beetroot.

Vegan Friendly Hyaluronic Acid (HA)– Hyaluronic acid is a substance within the body responsible for the hydration and suppleness of the skin. Its production decreases over time as a natural part of aging, causing the skin to become drier, thinner and looser. Plant sources with magnesium, zinc and vitamin C contain nutrients that support the production of hyaluronic acid and its presence in the skin. Good sources include bananas, avocados, figs, tropical fruits, leafy greens and broccoli, soy, and starchy root vegetables like sweet potatoes.

Aloe Soap Base

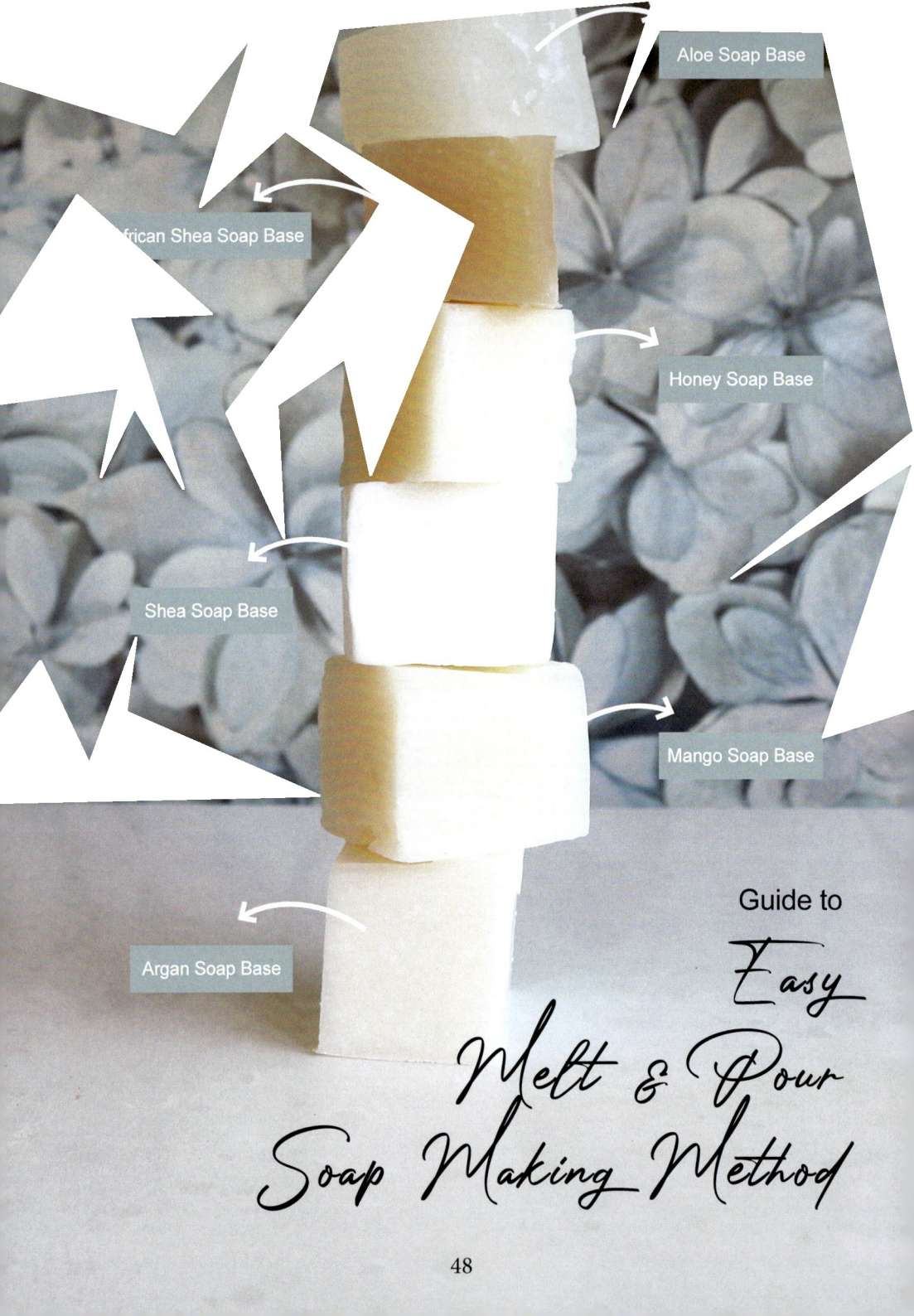

African Shea Soap Base

Honey Soap Base

Shea Soap Base

Mango Soap Base

Argan Soap Base

Guide to

Easy

Melt & Pour

Soap Making Method

Natural Soap Making has Never been Easier

I love working with all-natural melt and pour soap bases because it's quick, easy, safe and fun. The end product is loaded with skin-boosting nutrients and 100% effective — just check out our new soapsicle bars and honey waffles!

Product Versatility
There are so many types of melt and pour soap bases on the market like Shea, Mango, Argan, Honey and Aloe. Find the ones that fit your product type and you're off to a great start. You can create dozens of innovative and creative products with just one soap base, from shampoo bars and scalp bars to face bars to exfoliating shower bars. Just put on your marketing cap!

Easy as 1-2-3!
Simply cut your soap base into small pieces first, pop them into a Pyrex or pot and then melt it down in your double boiler. Once melted, you can add-in a few of your favourite raw ingredients like superfood powders, exfoliants, essential oils and clays. Create layers, create fun shapes and have fun.

Quick I Ready in 20 Minutes
Unlike cold-process soap, melt and pour does not require a whole production and curing process. Simply pop your molds into the fridge and allow the soap to set for about 25 minutes and it's ready to use.

No Specialized Equipment Needed
Unlike cold-process soap making, no specialized or expensive equipment is needed. I simply use a double boiler, silicone molds and a Pyrex. Invest in a few different silicone molds — they come in a variety of shapes and sizes and are easily washable and reusable. No special cutting tools required.

Chemical Free I Safe
Working with melt and pour is safe as no chemicals (like Lye) are required (no safety goggles required either). Today, there are so many melt and pour types on the market that are vegetable based, free from alcohol and harmful Lye, paraben free, PEG free and more. Just do your due diligence when sourcing melt and pour bases.

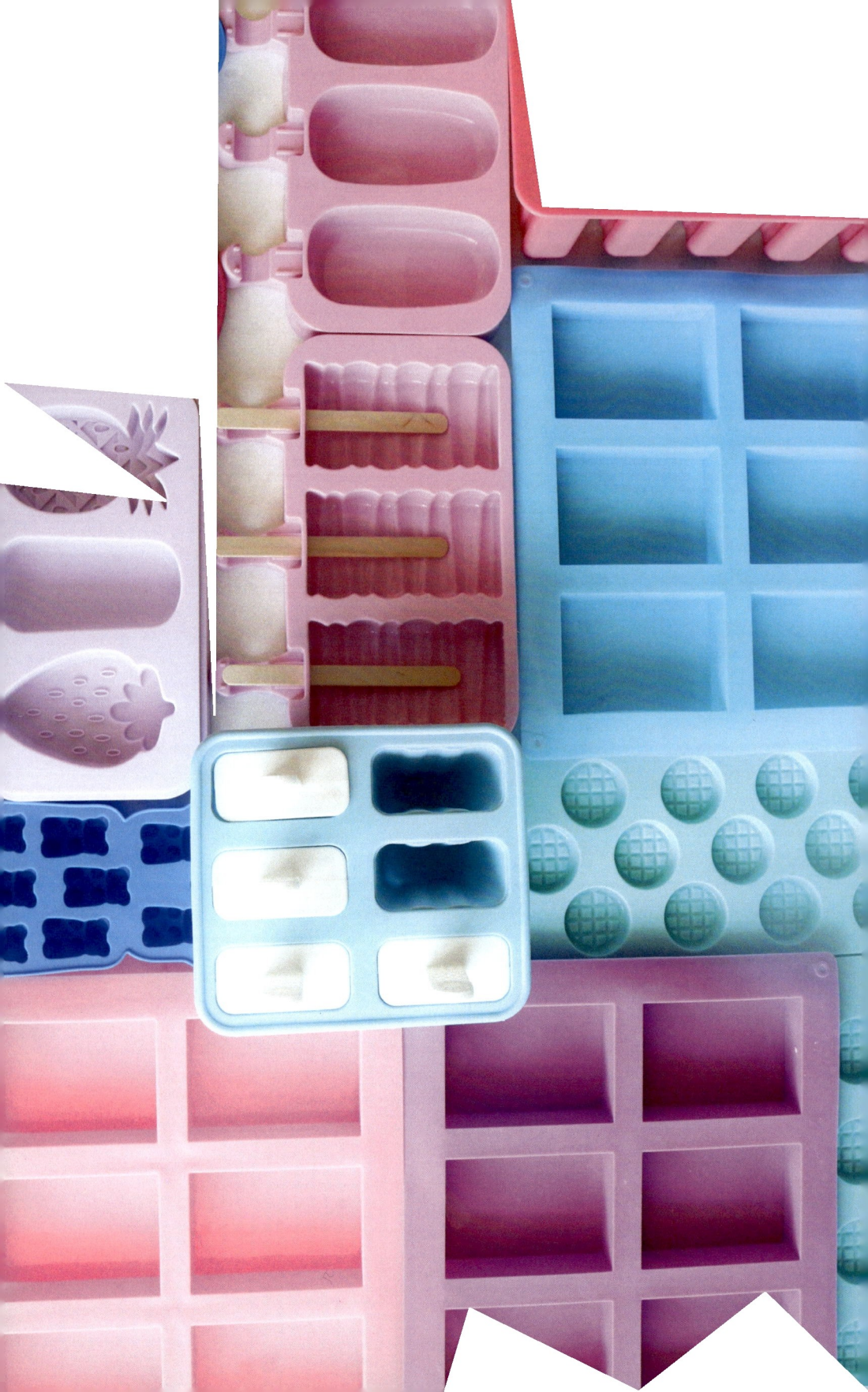

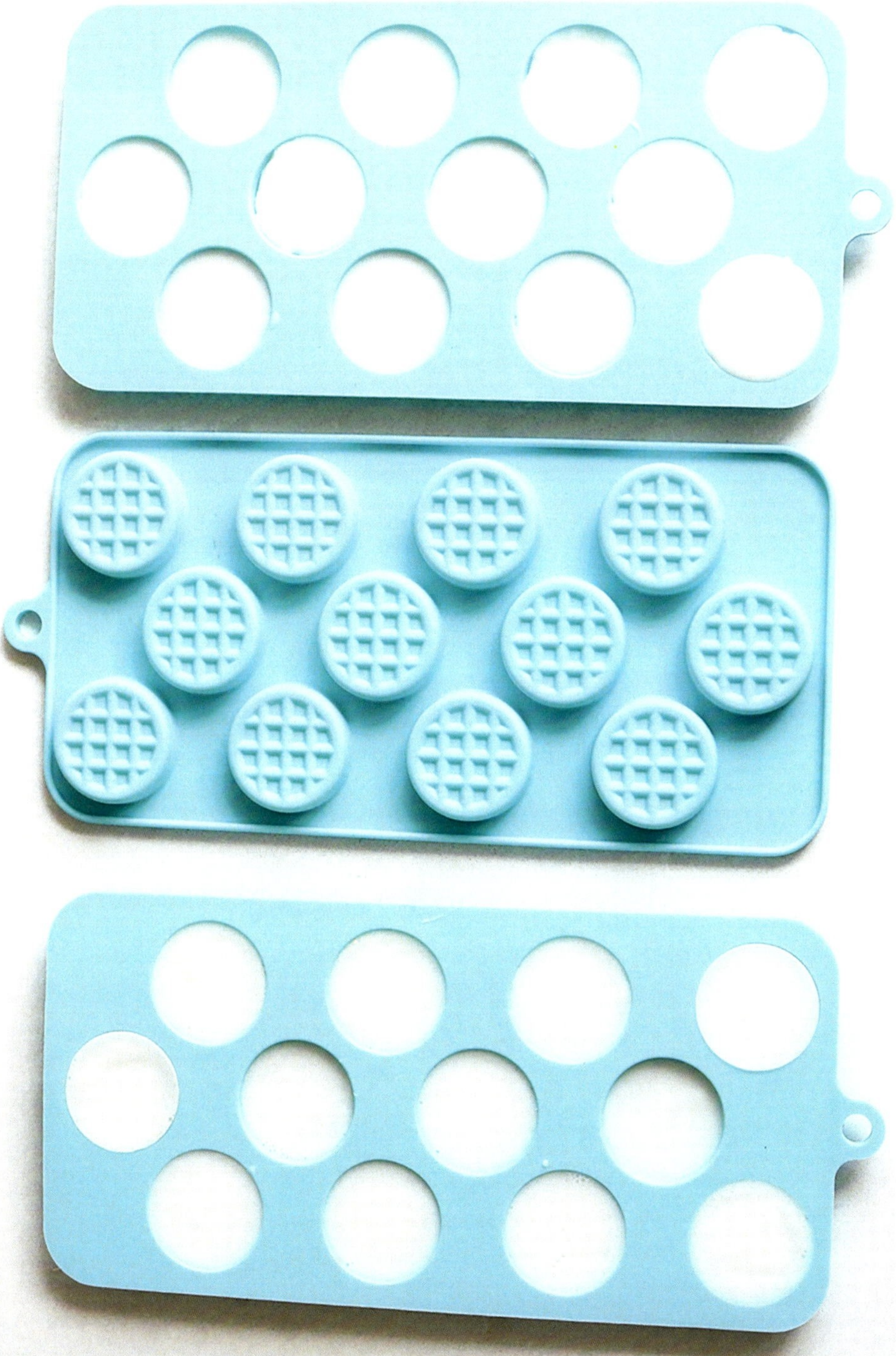

At-Home Self-care Skincare Rituals

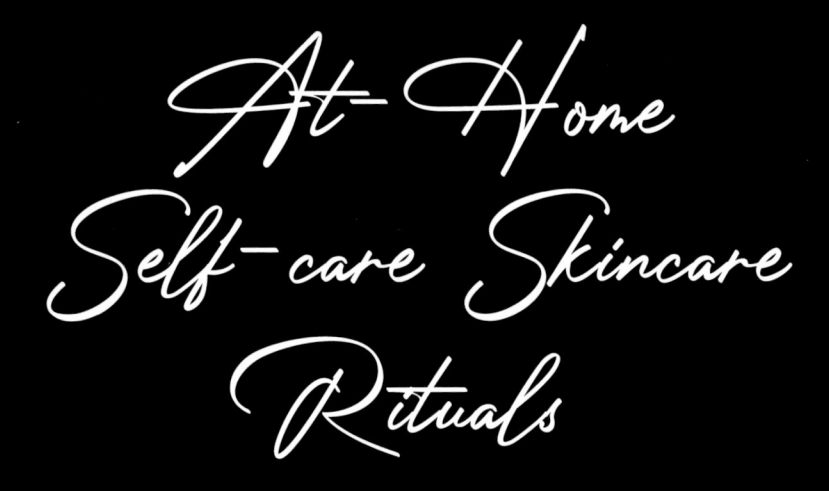

Create the Recipes | Build your own Rituals

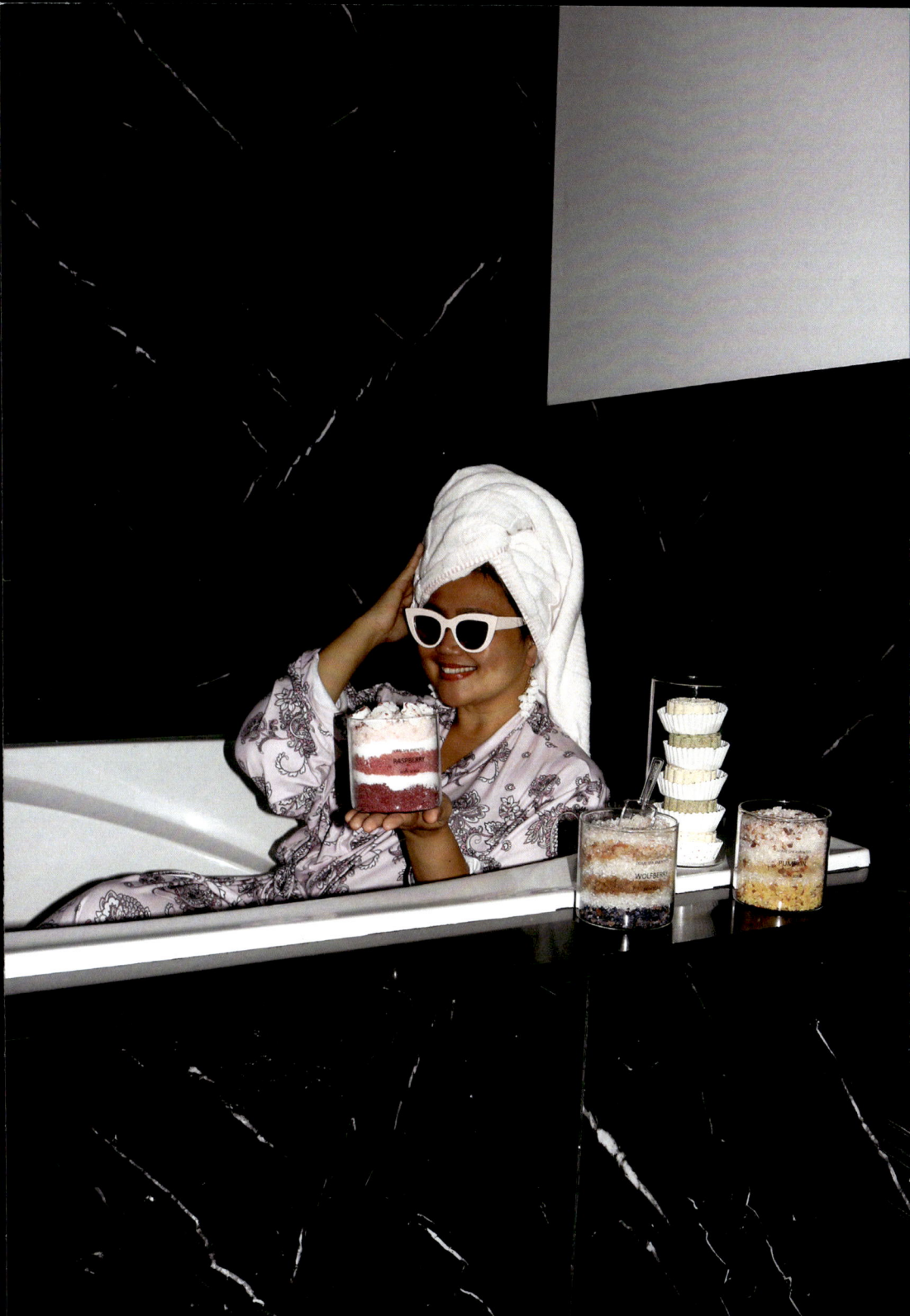

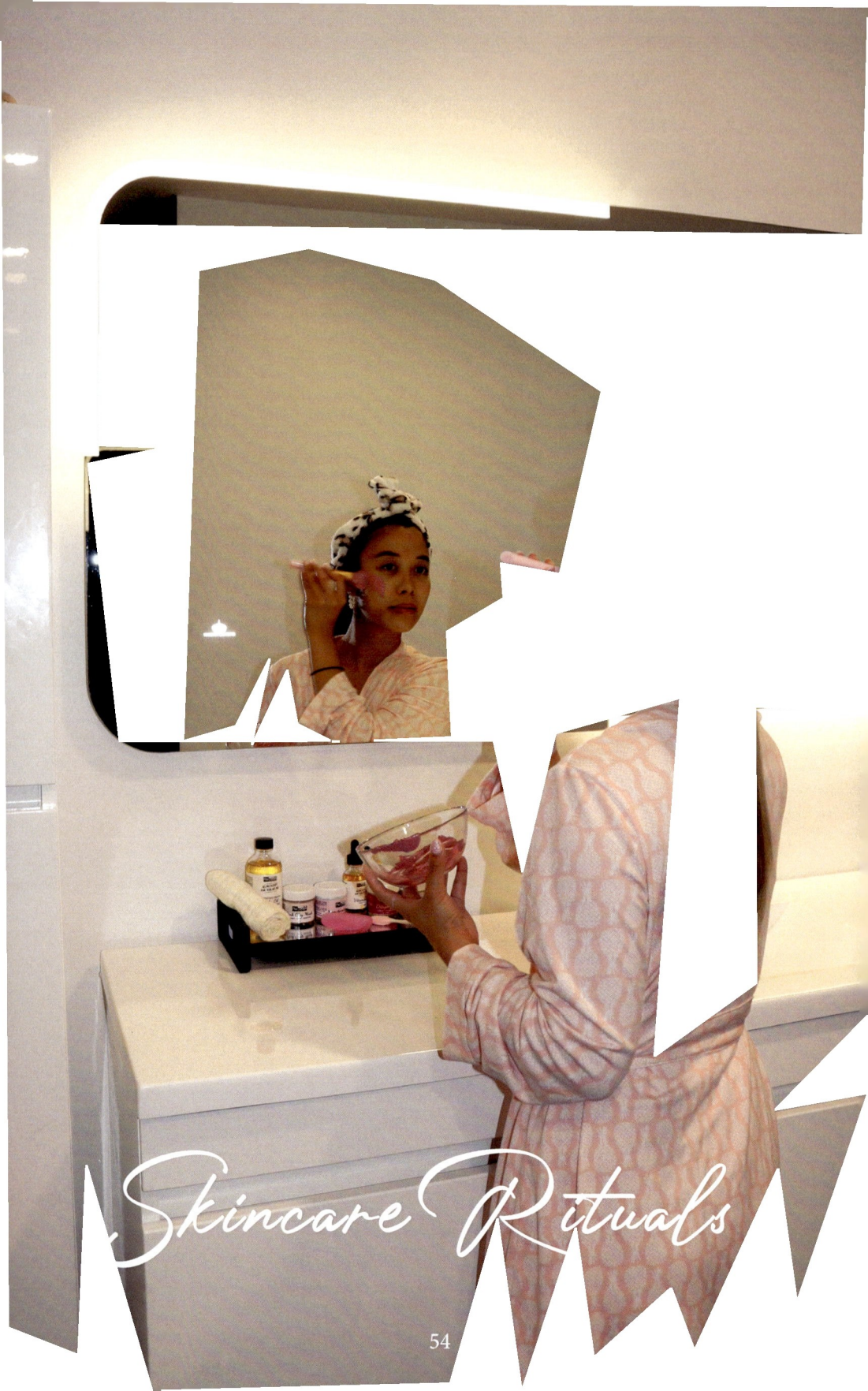

Skincare Rituals

Get Clear Skin: Build an Easy + Effective Skincare Routine

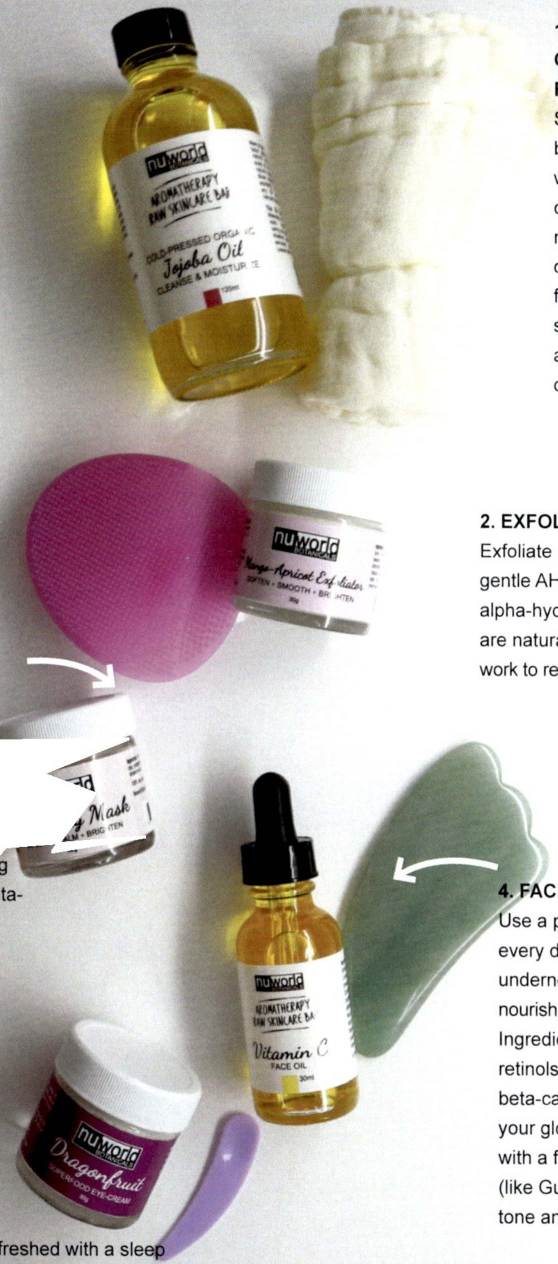

1. CLEANSE: HOT CLOTH CLEANSING RITUAL

Start and finish your day by cleansing the skin with oil (it's a thing, it's called the oil cleansing method). Oils naturally draw dirt and make-up from your pores to the surface. Gently wash it away with a soft cotton cloth.

2. EXFOLIATE

Exfoliate once a week with a gentle AHA fruit exfoliator. The alpha-hydroxy acids in superfruits are natural skin brighteners that work to reveal softer, smoother skin.

3. MASK

Treat your skin to a mineral clay mask (at least once a month). While the clays work to *[obscured]* and det*[obscured]* superfo*[obscured]* ingredie*[obscured]* addre*[obscured]* fro*[obscured]* mentation*[obscured]* lines *[obscured]*ss.

4. FACE OIL GLOW-UP

Use a plant-based face oil every day on clean skin (and underneath make-up) to nourish, hydrate and protect. Ingredients like natural source retinols, vitamin C and beta-carotene can amp up your glow game. Follow-up with a facial massage tool (like Gua Sha stone) to firm, tone and lift skin.

5. EYE CARE

Wake up looking refreshed with a sleep cream packed with eye-opening powerhouse ingredients like retinol, vitamins C and K.

Find all of these recipes under Skincare.

55

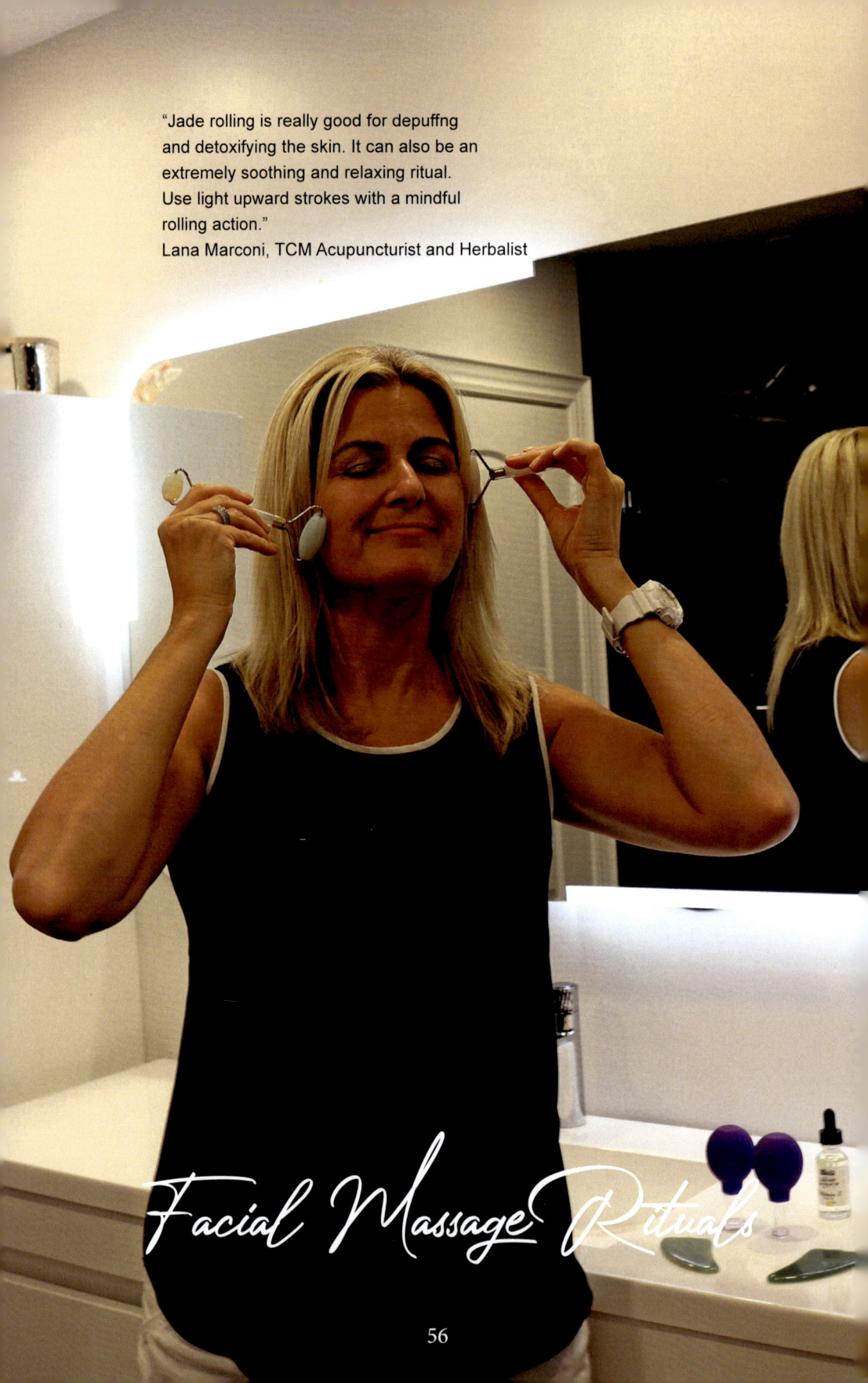

"Jade rolling is really good for depuffng and detoxifying the skin. It can also be an extremely soothing and relaxing ritual. Use light upward strokes with a mindful rolling action."
Lana Marconi, TCM Acupuncturist and Herbalist

Facial Massage Rituals

COLLAGEN BOOSTERS
The suction from facial cups (glass or silicone cups) promotes increased blood circulation, which may help relieve muscle tension, promote cell repair, and stimulate cells responsible for collagen production. It's also said to improve the flow of your "qi" (pronounced "chee"). Qi is a Chinese word meaning life force.

LAYER UP
Use your facial tools in conjunction with skincare products like this Vitamin Face Oil, which helps them glide over the skin easily (and helps the product penetrate further).

THE DEPUFFER
Jade rolling can be used daily to promote lymphatic drainage in the face. With the lymph system gently kicked into gear, excess fluid can be drained away, leaving you with less puffiness. Lift the skin with upward motions. Use on clean skin with a little face oil.

THE SCULPTOR
Gua Sha stones are positioned for giving the skin and tissue a "lift". Use these sculpting stones with a light press-and-sweep motion against lubricated skin.

GOOD VIBRATIONS
This 24k golden pulse facial massage is an anti-aging vibrating massage tool that helps increase blood circulation, tightness and fine lines and rejuvenate your skin.

LEARN THE TECHNIQUES WITH LANA'S EXPERT HOW-TO VIDEOS
For more information on how to use these skincare tools at home, please check out my sister Lana Marconi's online courses at Udemy.com: *Acupressure Face Massage, Cupping, Gua Sha and Jade Rolling. Cosmetic Acupuncture and Facial Rejuvenation.*

Bath Rituals

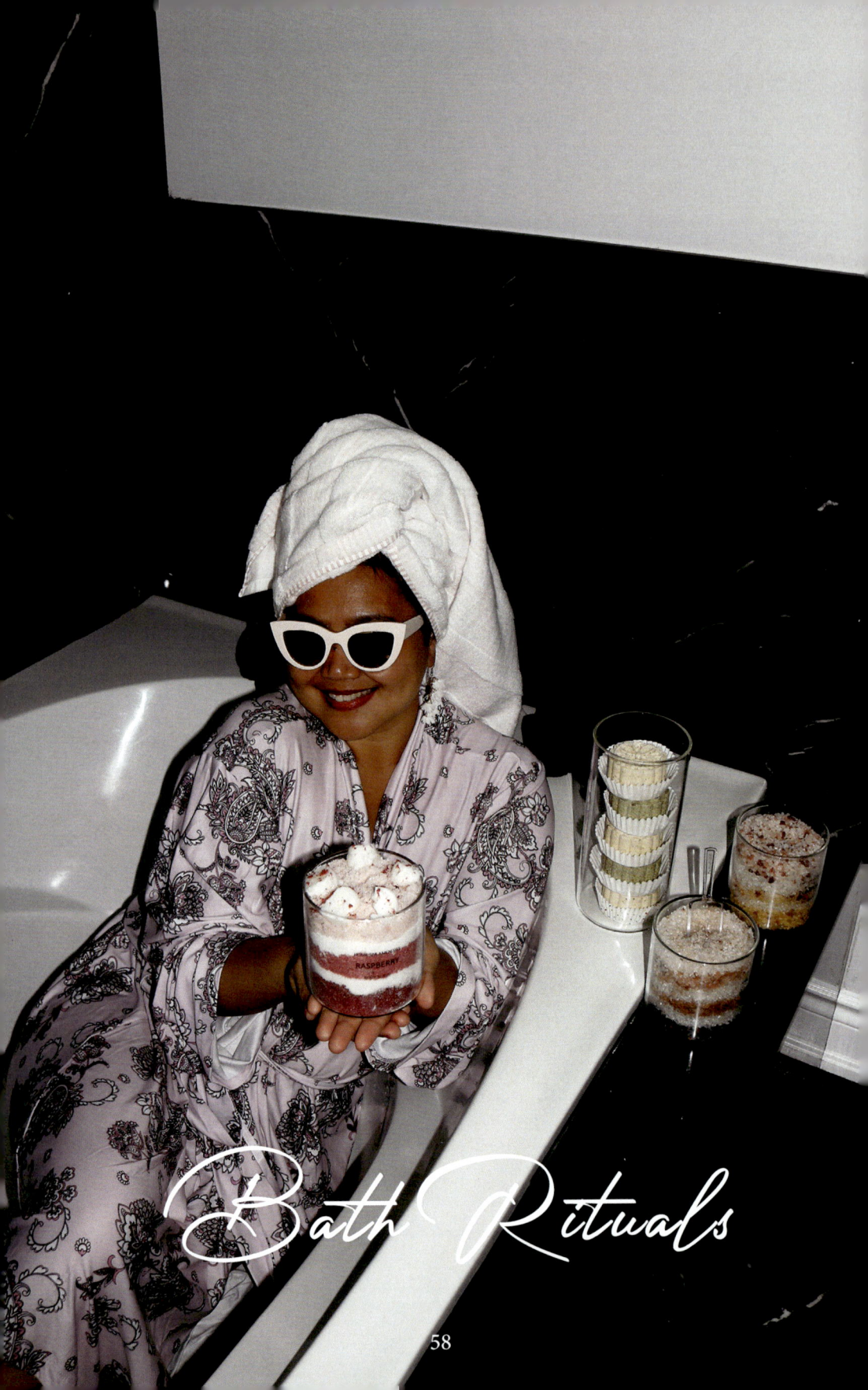

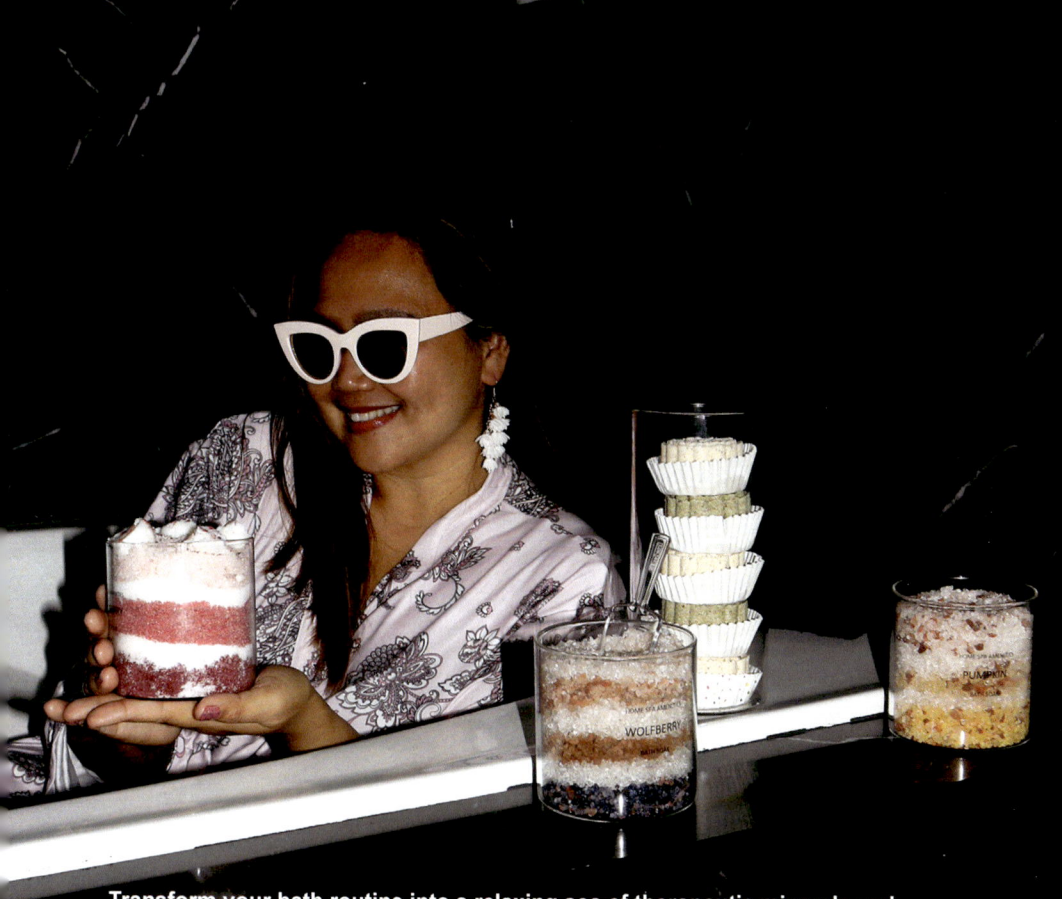

Transform your bath routine into a relaxing sea of therapeutic minerals and skin-boosting super fruit vitamins for glowing, radiant skin.

Superfruits like **Red Raspberry** are a hydrating ingredient packed with antioxidants that can help treat skin conditions like eczema and rashes. **Wolfberry** contains amino acids, which helps to improve the skin's tone and colour. **Pumpkin** is a great source of vitamin C, which helps improve skin texture and promote the production of collagen (thus improving skin tone and elasticity). **Mineral Sea Salts** are a powerful cleanser and can help rehydrate and restore depleted minerals.

Product (shown left to right): 1. Raspberry Mineral Salt-Balm Body Scrub. 2. Wolfberry Mineral Superfood Bath Soak. 3. Baked Superfood Mineral Bath Bombs. 4. Pumpkin Mineral Superfood Bath Soak. Find the recipes in *'DIY Bodycare Recipes.'*

Shower Rituals

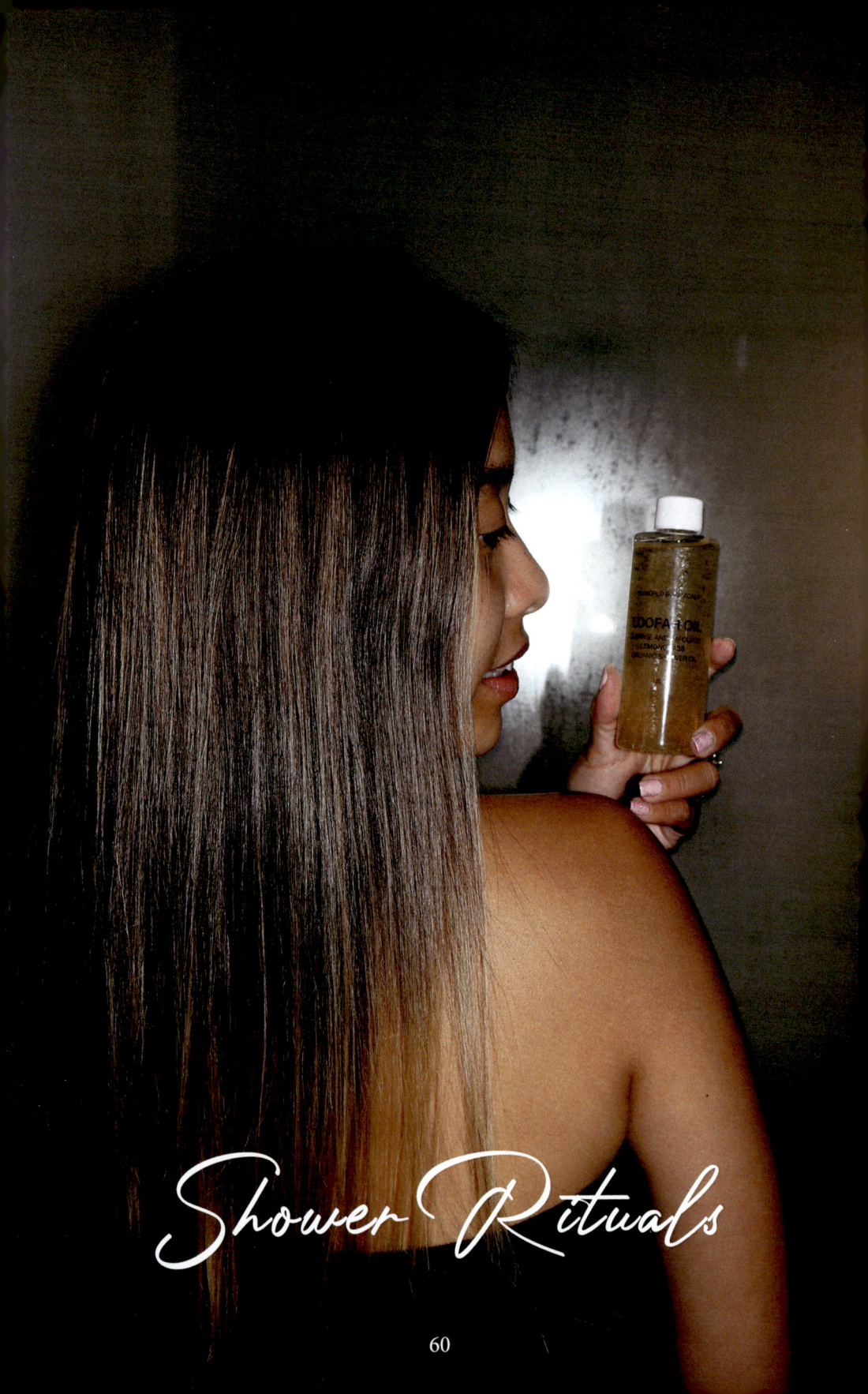

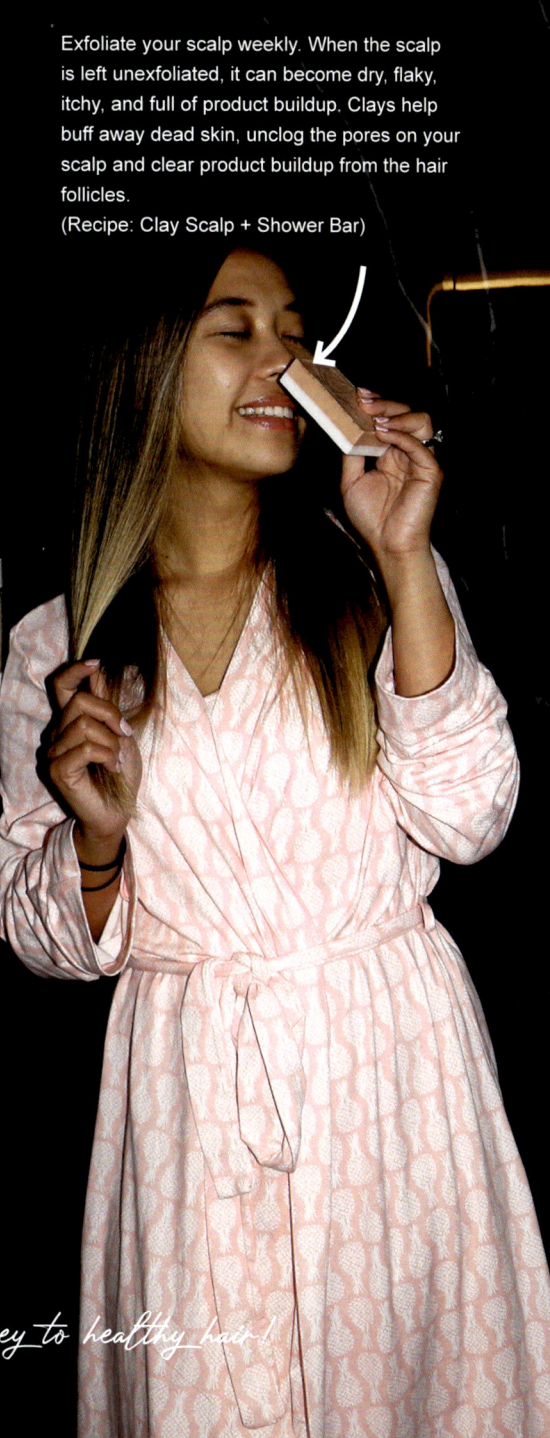

Exfoliate your scalp weekly. When the scalp is left unexfoliated, it can become dry, flaky, itchy, and full of product buildup. Clays help buff away dead skin, unclog the pores on your scalp and clear product buildup from the hair follicles.
(Recipe: Clay Scalp + Shower Bar)

Detox your scalp once a month with Dead Sea Salts and papaya extract to treat dandruff and other scalp conditions. The enzyme papain in papaya acts as a strong skin exfoliator and removes the dead cells.
(Recipe: Papaya Scalp + Body Scrub)

Cleanse the skin daily with hydrating, pore cleansing plant oils while gently exfoliating with raw loofah. Breathe in the transforming essential oils for an aromatherapy boost.
(Recipe: Loofah Shower Oils)

Flake-free scalps are the key to healthy hair!

Haircare Rituals

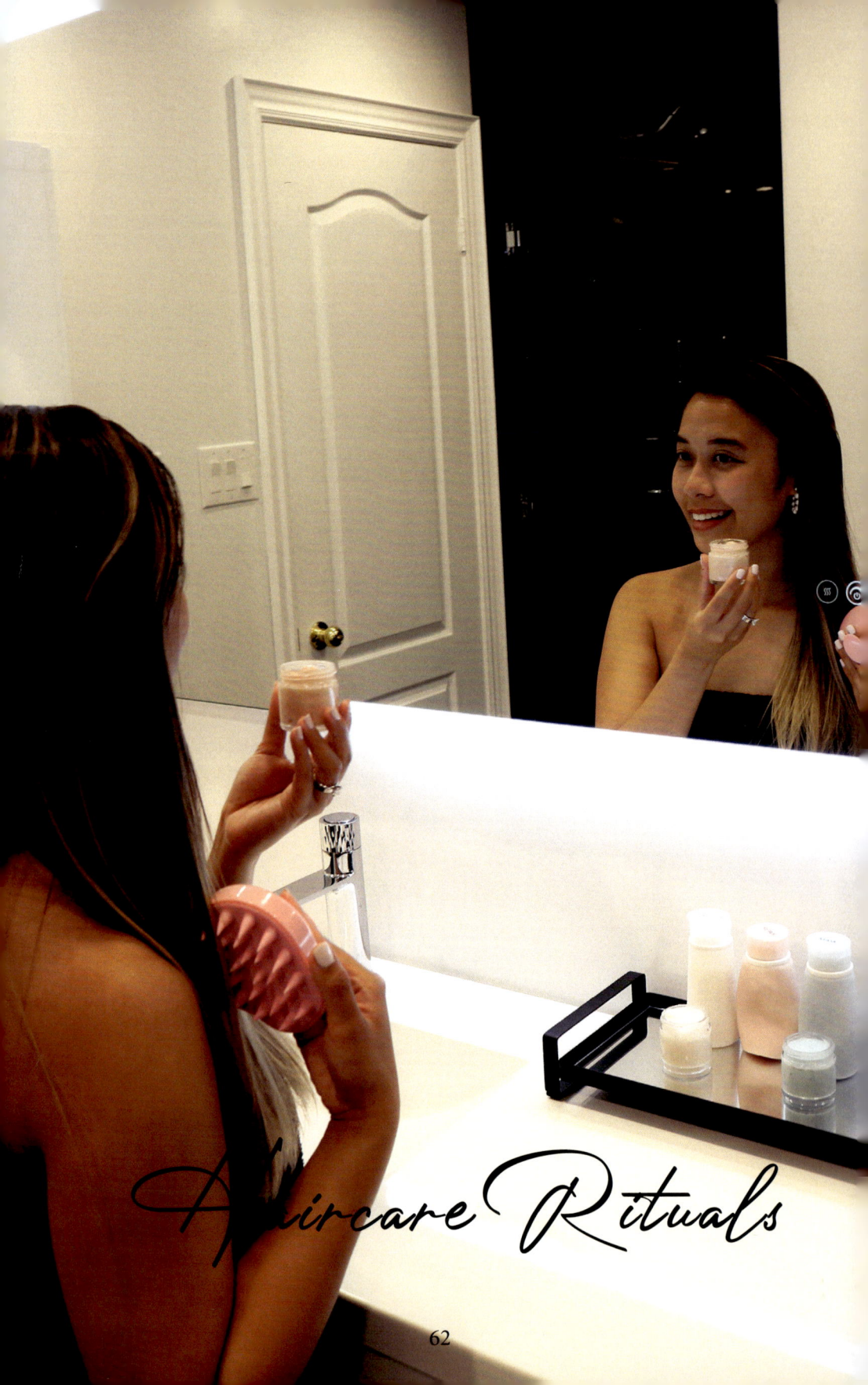

4-Step Haircare System

1. HUMECTANT HONEY MOISTURIZER
Your healthy hair moisturizer starts with power antioxidant butters like Murumuru and natural humectant superfood extracts like honey. As a natural humectant, honey maintains the hair's natural moisture balance, resulting in healthy, soft and stronger locks with a silky shine.
(Recipe: Honey Conditioner)

2. AT-HOME PROTEIN TREATMENT
Reinforce the exterior structure of your hair to improve texture, strength and appearance. Natural proteins and amino acids from red raspberry, bananas and broccoli seed are the hero ingredients. Apply this cream once a week, from roots to ends, on clean hair and detoxed scalp. Comb through and leave on for 10 minutes to fill in gaps in the cuticle, strengthen and smooth strands. Shampoo, condition.
(Recipe: Raspberry Repair)

SCALP MASSAGE TOOL
Stimulate the scalp and its follicles with this acupressure hair and scalp massage tool. Use it to comb products and serum, through from scalp to hair ends.

3. SLEEP HAIR MASK
Wake up to well-moisturized strands. This Blue clay overnight hair mask treatment penetrates your hair cuticles while you sleep, so you can wake up with smoother, softer and ridiculously shinier hair. Just apply and comb through your dry or wet hair before bed (slap on a hair wrap or shower cap if you like), and go to sleep. Rinse in the a.m.
(Recipe: Blue Clay Hair Mask)

4. SCALP TONIC TREATMENT
Handy dropper bottle provides on-the-spot application when your scalp begins to itch. Apply a few drops directly to scalp and massage it in. These cold-pressed organic oils are light and fast-drying.
(Recipe: Broccoli Scalp Serum)

EASY FLAKE-FREE LIPS
Kick things off by buffing away dry skin with this double-sided lip scrub tool and balmy lip scrub. Tiny beads of jojoba and gentle citric acid like lemon essential oil help smooth and soften your lips without stripping them dry. Scoop a tiny bit of the lip scrub onto the brush, rub it over your lips in a circular motion, and wipe your lips clean. Whip out this formula once a week and always follow up with a lip balm for extra hydration.
(Recipe: Butterfly Pea Lip Scrub)

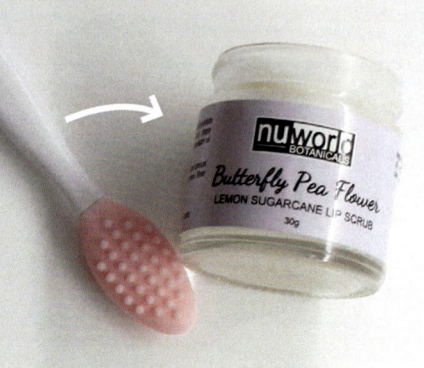

OVERNIGHT LIP MASK
The secret to softer, smoother lips in the morning? Condition and treat skin with nourishing plant oils like Camellia seed and hydrating lactic acid rich ingredients like Coconut Milk Powder and Apple Cider Vinegar. Try this lip mask recipe once a week before bed.
(Recipe: Lactic Acid Apple Sleep Lip Mask)

EVERYTHING BALM
Coat lips in a blanket of soothing (and vegan) HA-packed ingredients like Soy butter and bananas. It's extra thick and satisfying to use especially if you're struggling with severely dry or cracked lips.
(Recipe: HA Banana Face Balm)

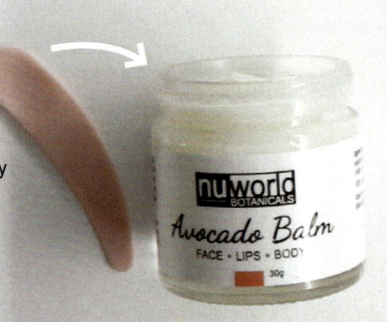

Lip Care Rituals

Sweet Dreams Aromatherapy

The purpose of a bedtime routine is to relax and de-stress. On nights when you need extra help loosening up and calming down, a little Aromatherapy does the body good. Essential oils known to promote calm and relaxation include Lavender, Chamomile, Rose and Marjoram.

SWEET DREAMS ROLL-ON
Just before bed, massage this rollerball sleep elixir onto your skin. Breath in the transforming essential oils for an overall sense of restoration and well-being. Enjoy a good nights rest.
(Recipe: Sweet Dreams Roll-on)

SWEET DREAMS BODY, BATH AND HAIR OIL
After your bath or shower, follow up with a moisturizing blend of plant oils like camellia seed and hemp seed. Add calming essential oils to promote sleep.
(Recipe: Vitamin C Body Oil)

SWEET DREAMS AROMATHERAPY BUTTER
Butter up dry skin with a hydrating blend of butters and plant oils. Add calming essential oils like Lavender and Marjoram for sleep.
(Recipe: Superfood Body Cream)

Bedtime Rituals

Guest Amenities

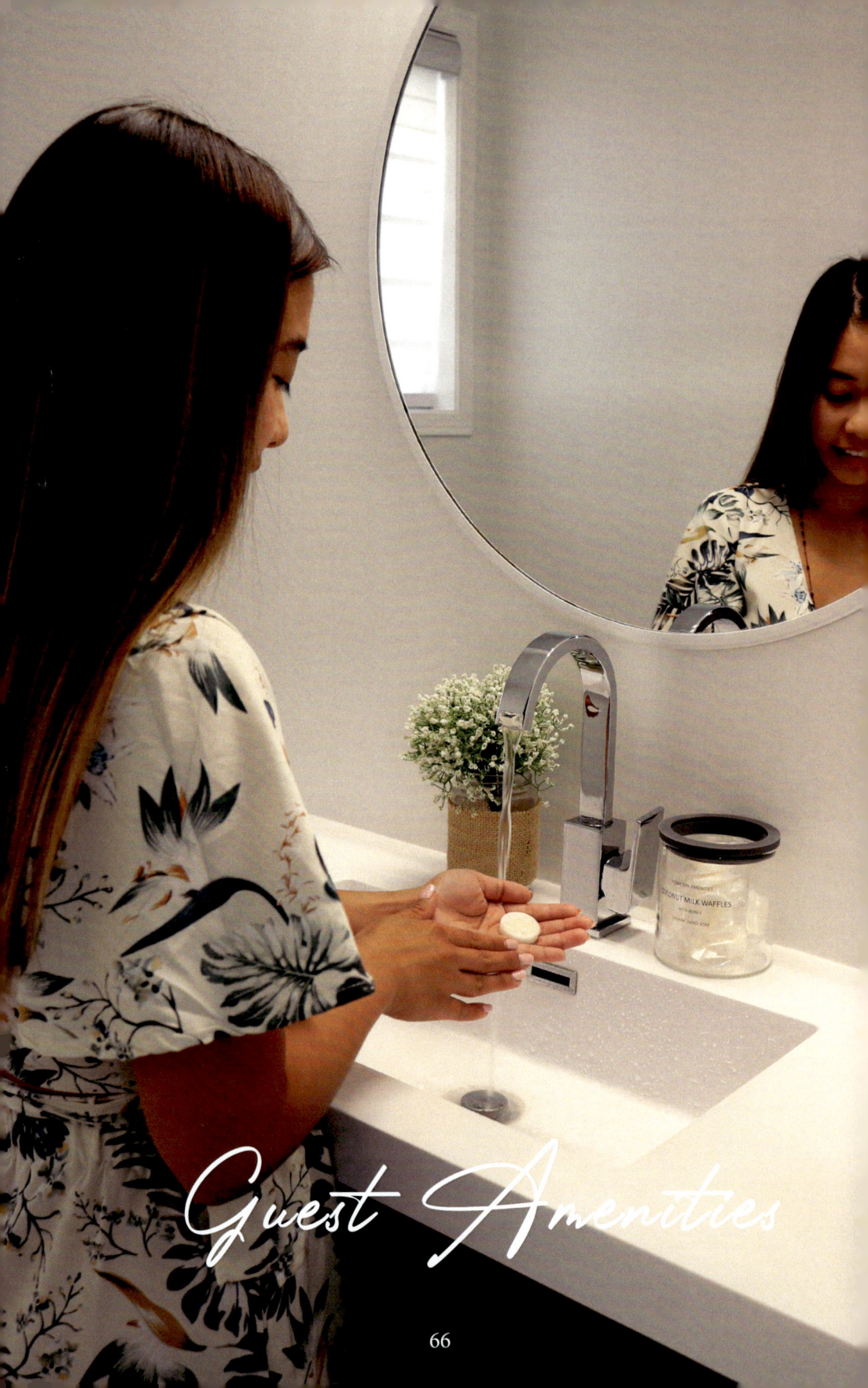

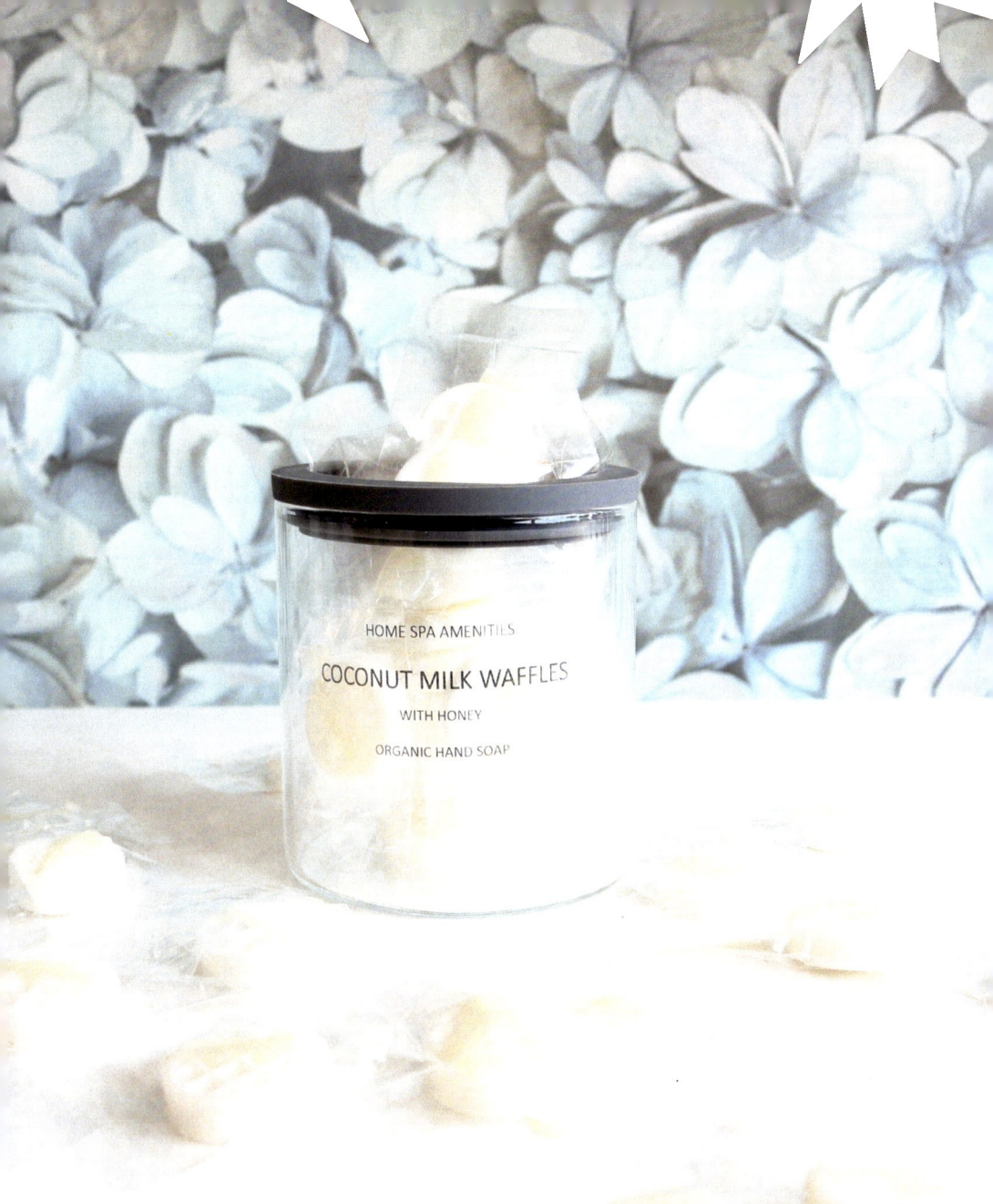

Treat your house guests to luxurious spa-at-home treats. These pretty one-time use waffle soaps can be individually wrapped and left out on your powder room counter. The lactic acid in coconut milk is extremely softening and soothing on dry itchy skin. Honey drizzle adds natural antibacterial properties. We wrap our soaps in eco-bags made from wood pulp. No plastic here!

(Recipe: Coconut Milk Waffle Hand Soaps)

Diy Superfood Skincare Recipes

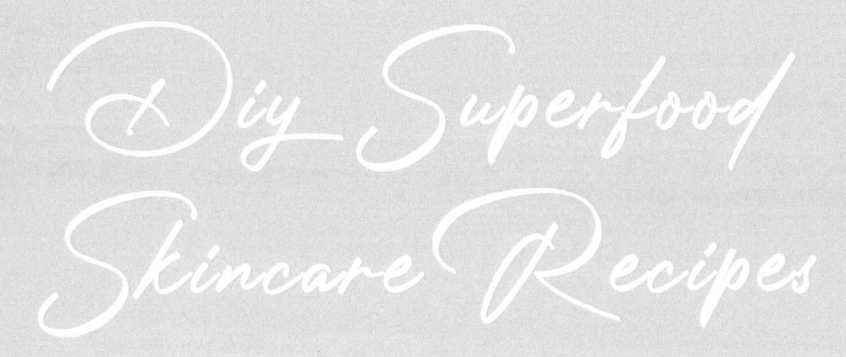

Get your glow-up!

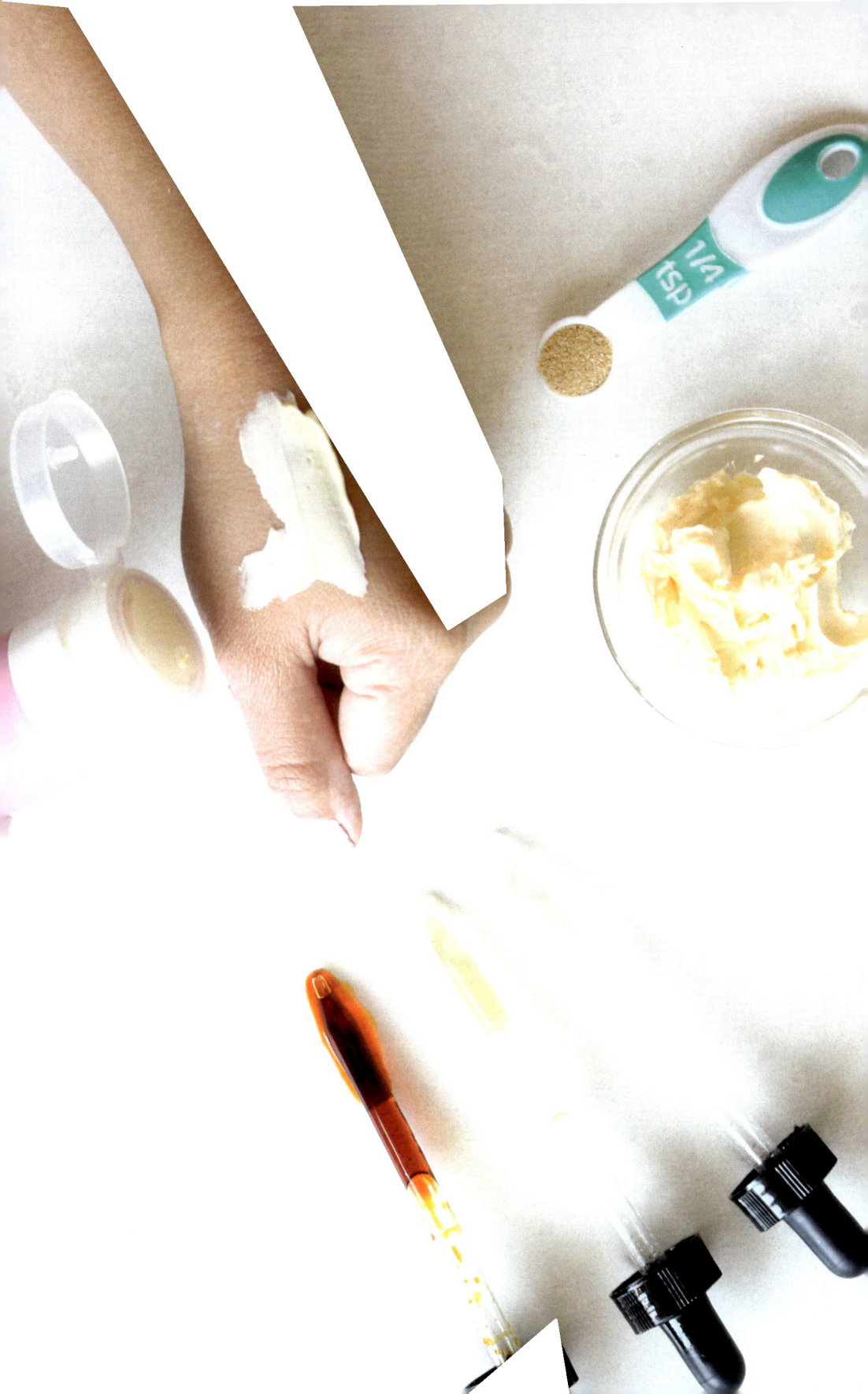

Salicylic Blueberry Oil Face Wash

This fast-absorbing natural-source salicylic acid oil cleanser is the best option for breakout-prone skin. Blueberry oil is naturally high in salicylates (the salt of salicylic acid) that helps minimize pores, open and clean clogged pores and aid against bacteria that causes breakout. Grape seed oil has antibacterial properties and omega fatty acids (like linolenic acid) that can help clear up acne. Removes make-up like a charm.

Raw Ingredients:

50 ml grape seed oil
50 ml blueberry oil
10 ml broccoli oil
5 ml fractionated coconut oil
5 ml raspberry oil

Kitchen Tools:

You will need a funnel and a bottle.

Recipe Prep Time

Prep Time: 5 minutes
Set Time: 5 minutes
Qty: 120 ml bottle

Hot Cloth Cleansing Ritual: Apply a quarter-sized amount of oil over dry skin and massage in circular motions. Wet a cotton-organic face cloth in warm water, and wring it out. Press cloth into skin, hold for 30 seconds to lift dirt from pores. Wipe away. Repeat for a double cleanse if needed.

Method:

1. Fill bottle with carrier oils.
2. Close cap and shake bottle well.

Vitamin C Creamy Exfoliating Cleanser

Brighten up! This cleanser uses multiple exfoliating agents to smooth and polish the skin's surface including lime powder and fig seeds. Natural source vitamin C comes from carrot oil and sea buckthorn oil, while Shea butter hydrates and delivers vitamin E to the skin.

Raw Ingredients:

20 g shea butter
10 g cupuacu butter
20 ml hemp seed oil
5 ml carrot oil
110 ml distilled water
1/2 tsp lime superfood powder
1/2 tsp sea buckthorn superfood powder
1/4 tsp fig seeds exfoliant
15 g emulsifying wax
5 ml natural preservative (Leucidal® Liquid Complete)
5 drops sea buckthorn oil
2 drops vitamin E (MT-50)

Kitchen Tools:

You will need a double boiler, two small pots, scale, whisk, piping bag, measuring spoons, two beakers, electric mixer and a silicone squeezy bottle.

Recipe Prep Time

Prep Time: 15 minutes
Set Time: 30 minutes
Qty: 120 g bottle

Method:

1. In a double boiler, gradually melt the shea butter, cupuacu butter and emulsifying wax (pot 1).
2. Once melted, add in the hemp seed and carrot oil and whisk (pot 1).
3. In a SEPARATE pot (pot 2), heat up the distilled water and add the superfood extract powders. Whisk.
4. Remove Pot 1 from heat and pour into a clean dry beaker (Beaker 1).
5. Remove Pot 2 from heat and pour into a SEPARATE beaker (Beaker 2).
6. Slowly pour beaker 2 into beaker 1 while whisking (this must be done gradually so take about 2 minutes to complete this step).
7. Leave the mixture in the beaker and out on the counter to cool for about 3 minutes, and then add in the natural preservative, sea buckthorn oil and vitamin E. Mix well with a whisk.
8. Pop the beaker into the fridge for about 30 minutes or until semi-solid.
9. You can then fluff it up with an electric hand mixer (add your fig seeds in here) and then transfer the cream to a bottle using a piping bag.

Mango Melting Milk Cleanser Balm & Make-up Remover

This luxe balm quickly turns to an oil upon contact with your skin. Cleanses while drawing moisture to the skin. Rich with vitamins A, E and lactic acid. Leaves skin feeling ultra-soft and supple and gently removes make-up. Perfect for sensitive and mature dry skin.

Raw Ingredients:

20 g mango butter
5 g shea butter
1/4 tsp organic coconut superfood powder
5 drops meadowfoam oil
5 drops calendula oil
1 drop sea buckthorn oil

Kitchen Tools:

You will need a double boiler, one small pot, scale, whisk, measuring spoons, beaker and a jar.

Recipe Prep Time

Prep Time: 15 minutes
Set Time: 15 minutes
Qty: 30 g jar

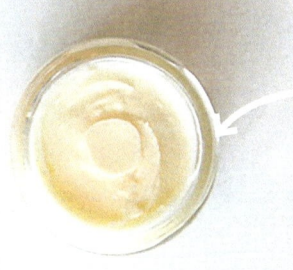

Ritual: This luxe balm quickly melts to an oil upon contact with your skin. Massage into skin using circular motions; press and rinse with a soft cotton cloth.

Method:

1. In a double boiler, gently melt down the shea and mango butter.
2. Add in the carrier oils (meadowfoam, calendula).
3. Add in the superfood extract powder and whisk well.
4. Transfer into a clean dry beaker and add in the sea buckthorn oil.
5. Pour the mixture into a clean dry jar (put lid on tightly).
6. Pop in the jar in the fridge for about 15 minutes, to set faster.

Lactic Acid Apple Hydrating Mask

This gentle lactic acid rich mask smooths and brightens dull and dry skin by lightly exfoliating dead skin cells. Key superfood ingredients coconut milk and apple cider vinegar help to improve skin's texture through exfoliation, while keeping the skin moisturized.

Raw Ingredients:

25 g rhassoul clay
25 g pink clay
1 tsp kaolin white clay
1 tsp organic coconut powder
1/4 tsp lime superfood powder
1/4 tsp lemon superfood powder
1/4 tsp apple cider superfood powder

Kitchen Tools:

You will need measuring spoons and a jar.

Recipe Prep Time

Prep Time: 5 minutes
Set Time: 5 minutes
Qty: 60 g jar

How to Use: In a separate bowl, mix 1 tsp of clay with 1 tsp of water to form a thin paste. Apply a thin layer to your face (avoiding eyes) for five minutes then rinse with a warm cloth. Follow up with a face oil.

Method:

1. Fill jar with clays.
2. Add in the superfood extracts.
3. Top up with more kaolin white clay until jar is full.
4. Shake well and combine before use.

Salicylic Purple Potato Acne Mask

As part of your acne treatment, decongest the skin and refine skin tone and texture with an array of natural salicylic ingredients like white willow bark and sweet potato. Follow up this mask treatment with a hydrating face oil to balance out the skin's pH.

Raw Ingredients:

20 g purple clay
10 g beige kaolin clay
1 tsp kaolin white clay
1 tsp sweet potato superfood powder
1/2 tsp white willow superfood powder
1/4 tsp beet root superfood powder

Kitchen Tools:

You will need measuring spoons and a jar.

Recipe Prep Time

Prep Time: 5 minutes
Set Time: 5 minutes
Qty: 30 g jar

Tip: Keep this jar dry and take out a scoop as needed. There is enough mask in this jar to last approximately 2-3 months if you mask once a week.

Method:

1. Fill jar with clays.
2. Add in the superfood powders.
3. Top up jar with more kaolin white clay until jar is full.
4. Shake well and combine before use.

Glycolic Papaya-C Bright Face Mask

This recipe is chock-full of tropical AHAs that exfoliates the skin and turn over cells to give it that luminous glow. Turmeric pairs with pineapple and papaya enzymes to fight hyperpigmentation and dullness. Evening out the skin tone and can help lessen the appearance of superficial scars and hyperpigmentation.

Raw Ingredients:

40 g french yellow clay
1 tsp white kaolin clay
1 tsp papaya superfood powder
1 tsp pineapple superfood powder
1/2 tsp honey superfood powder
1/4 tsp turmeric superfood powder

Kitchen Tools:

You will need measuring spoons and a jar.

Recipe Prep Time

Prep Time: 5 minutes
Set Time: 5 minutes
Qty: 60 g jar

Tip: Instead of mixing with water each time, change it up! Try adding your favourite floral water (tea tree, lemongrass, rose) or even apple cider vinegar for instance.

Method:

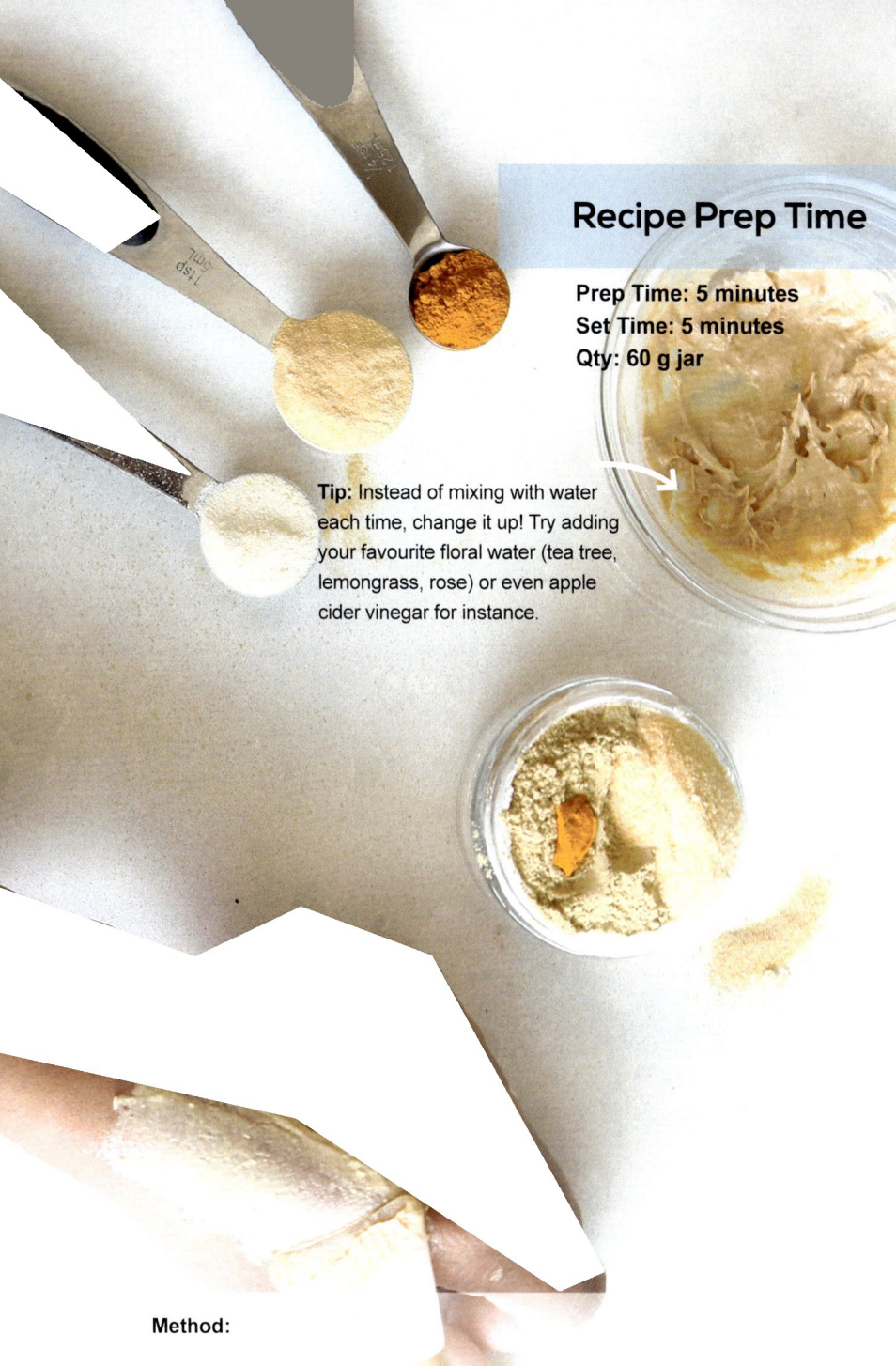

1. Fill jar with clays.
2. Add in the superfood powders.
3. Top up jar with more kaolin white clay until jar is full.
4. Shake well and combine before use.

Citric Tangerine-C Powder Exfoliator

An exfoliating powder is a good intro to exfoliating acids, as the contact time with the skin is shorter than with a mask and can be targeted to areas that need exfoliation the most. Tangerine powder is rich with citric acid, that helps dissolve skin-clogging debris. Vitamin C ingredients, including blueberry powder and ascorbic acid ensure a healthy after-glow.

Raw Ingredients:

20 g moroccan rhassoul clay
1 tsp kaolin white clay
1 tsp coffee exfoliant
1/2 tsp tangerine superfood powder
1/2 tsp vitamin C (ascorbic acid) powder
1/4 tsp blueberry superfood powder

Kitchen Tools:

You will need measuring spoons and a jar.

Recipe Prep Time

Prep Time: 5 minutes
Set Time: 5 minutes
Qty: 30 g jar

Tip: Pair the exfoliator with a soft silicone face massage tool. It helps promote circulation and helps with exfoliation of dead cells.

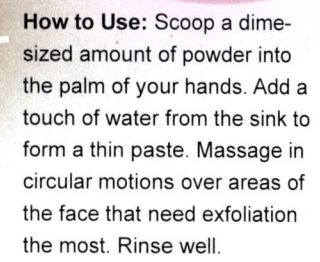

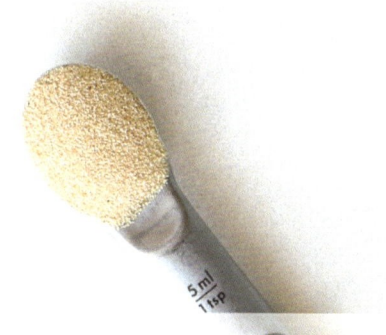

How to Use: Scoop a dime-sized amount of powder into the palm of your hands. Add a touch of water from the sink to form a thin paste. Massage in circular motions over areas of the face that need exfoliation the most. Rinse well.

Method:

1. Fill jar with clays.
2. Add in the superfood extracts and vitamin C powder.
3. Add your coffee exfoliant.
4. Top up with more kaolin white clay until jar is full.
5. Shake well and combine before use.

Vitamin K– Apricot Dark Circle Face Oil

This anti-aging powerhouse is loaded with powerful antioxidants like beta-carotene and vitamins C and K, which can stimulate tissue renewal and help decrease dark circles and puffiness.

Raw Ingredients:

20 ml apricot kernel oil
5 ml olive oil
4 ml carrot oil
5 drops lavender essential oil (optional)
2 drops sea buckthorn oil

Kitchen Tools:

You will need a dropper, funnel and a bottle.

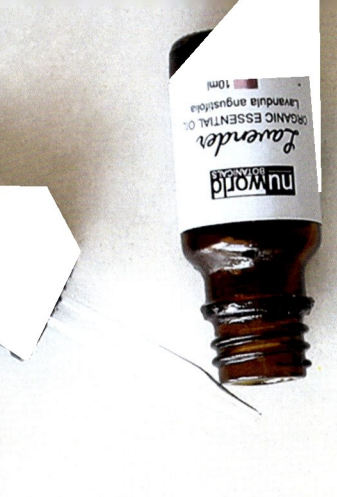

Recipe Prep Time

Prep Time: 5 minutes
Set Time: 5 minutes
Qty: 30 ml bottle

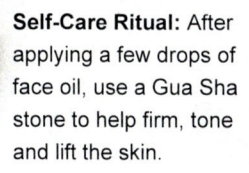

Self-Care Ritual: After applying a few drops of face oil, use a Gua Sha stone to help firm, tone and lift the skin.

Method:

1. Fill bottle with carrier oils.
2. Add in the essential oil (optional) and sea buckthorn oil.
3. Top up with more carrier oil if needed.
4. Close cap and shake well before use.

HA Hydrating Green Veggie Serum

Take your healthy green veggies! Broccoli contains high levels of vitamin A, C and magnesium which increases the amount of hyaluronan in the skin, elevating moisture levels and encouraging skin health. Avocado oil may help speed up skin repair and improve eczema. All skin types can benefit from this green smoothie concoction.

Raw Ingredients:

15 ml broccoli oil
5 ml avocado oil
5 ml raspberry oil
5 ml grape seed oil
8 drops rose essential oil (optional)

Kitchen Tools:

You will need a small funnel, dropper and a bottle.

Recipe Prep Time

Prep Time: 5 minutes
Set Time: 5 minutes
Qty: 30 ml bottle

Tip: Chill your face roller in the refrigerator and use it in the morning for a more refreshing face massage. This can help reduce puffiness after sleeping and help you to feel more awake.

Method:

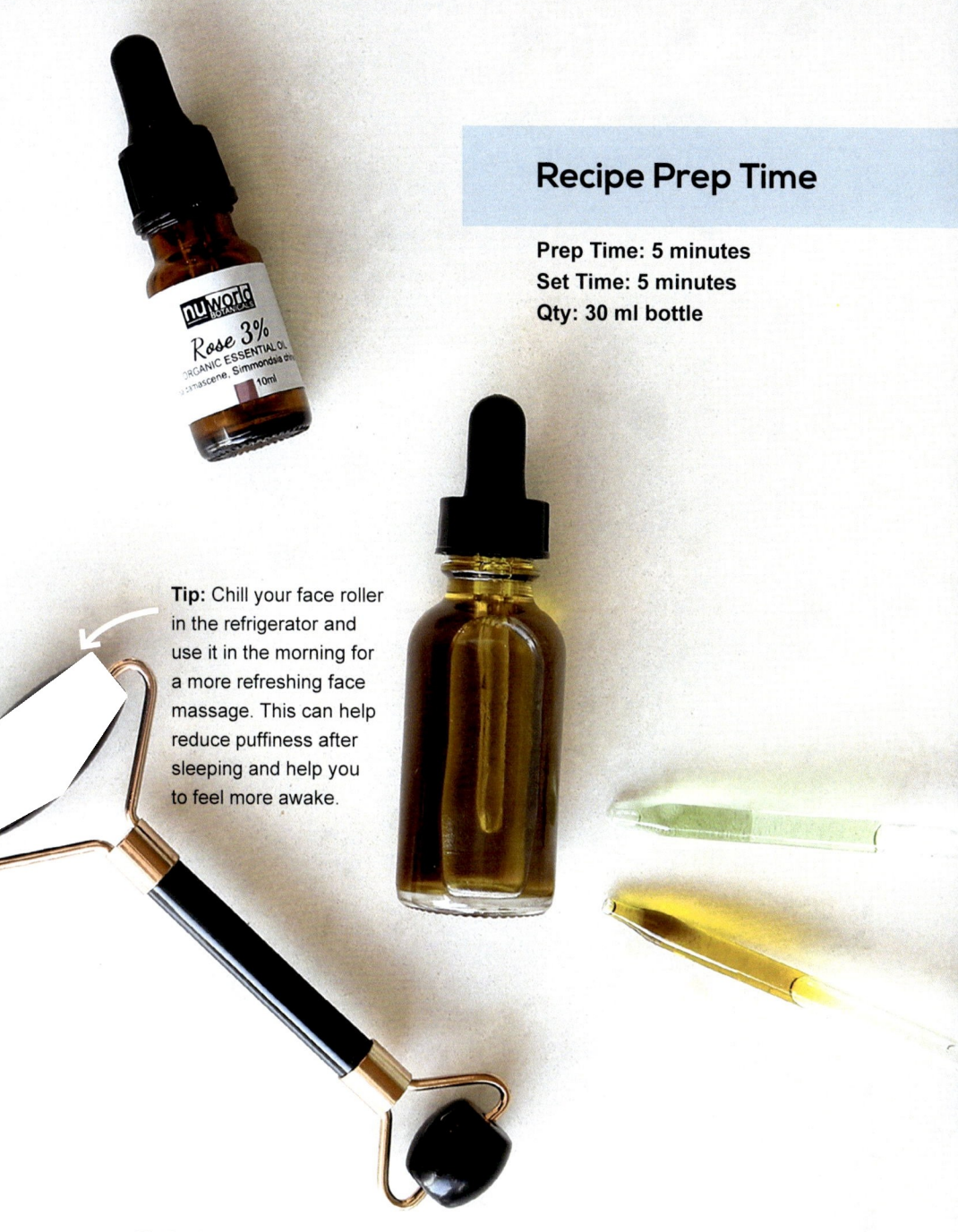

1. Fill bottle with carrier oils.
2. Add in the essential oil (optional).
3. Top up with more carrier oil if needed.
4. Close cap and shake well before use.

Glycolic Fruits Hyperpigmentation Face Oil

This superfruit mix is a concentrated blend of delicious fruit brighteners and vitamin C extracts, to help promote firmer and smoother skin. Alpha Hydroxy Acids (AHA) renew skin cells to reveal a younger and fresher skin appearance.

Raw Ingredients:

20 ml superfruit mix oil (sugar cane, orange, lemon fruit, sugar maple)
5 ml blueberry oil
5 ml pomegranate oil
8 drops bergamot essential oil (optional)

Kitchen Tools:

You will need a dropper, funnel and a bottle.

Recipe Prep Time

Prep Time: 5 minutes
Set Time: 5 minutes
Qty: 30 ml bottle

Self-Care Ritual: Pair your facial oil with beautiful glass facial cups for the ultimate glow-up!

Method:

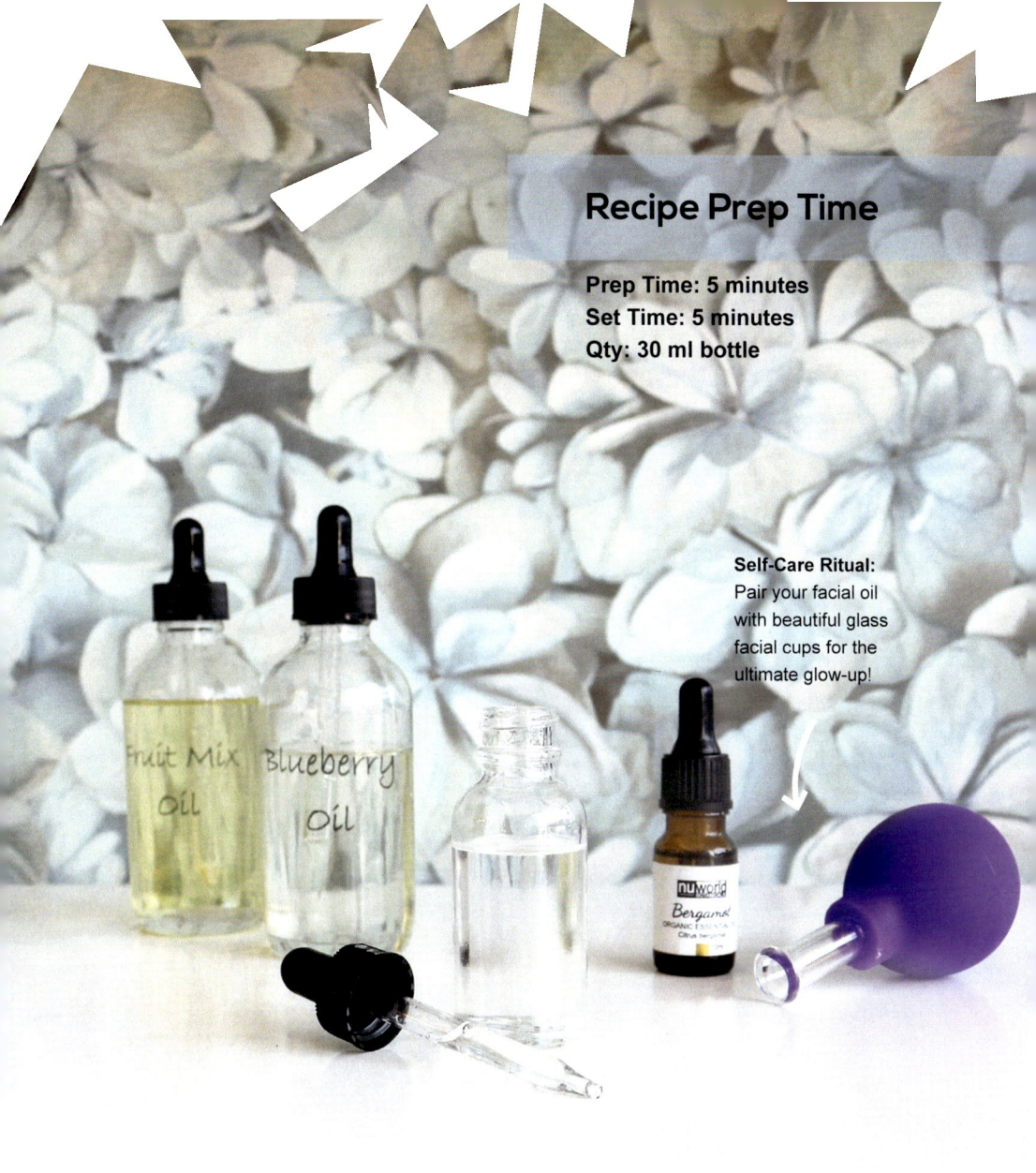

1. Fill bottle with carrier oils.
2. Add in the essential oil (optional).
3. Top up with more carrier oil if needed.
4. Close cap and shake well before use.

Pineapple Enzyme Sleep Cream

Glycolic acid from pineapple regenerates collagen, evens out the skin tone and can help lessen the appearance of superficial scars and hyperpigmentation. Layer it on face at night so the regenerating glycolic acid can get to work.

Raw Ingredients:

20 g shea butter
10 g cocoa butter
20 ml argan oil
5 ml jojoba oil
110 ml distilled water
1/2 tsp pineapple superfood powder
1/2 tsp papaya superfood powder
15 g emulsifying wax
5 ml natural preservative (Leucidal Liquid Complete)
10 drops geranium essential oil (optional)
2 drops vitamin E (MT-50)
2 drops sea buckthorn oil

Kitchen Tools:

You need a double boiler, two small pots, scale, whisk, spatula, measuring spoons, two beakers, electric mixer and a jar.

Recipe Prep Time

Prep Time: 15 minutes
Set Time: 30 minutes
Qty: 120 g jar

Method:

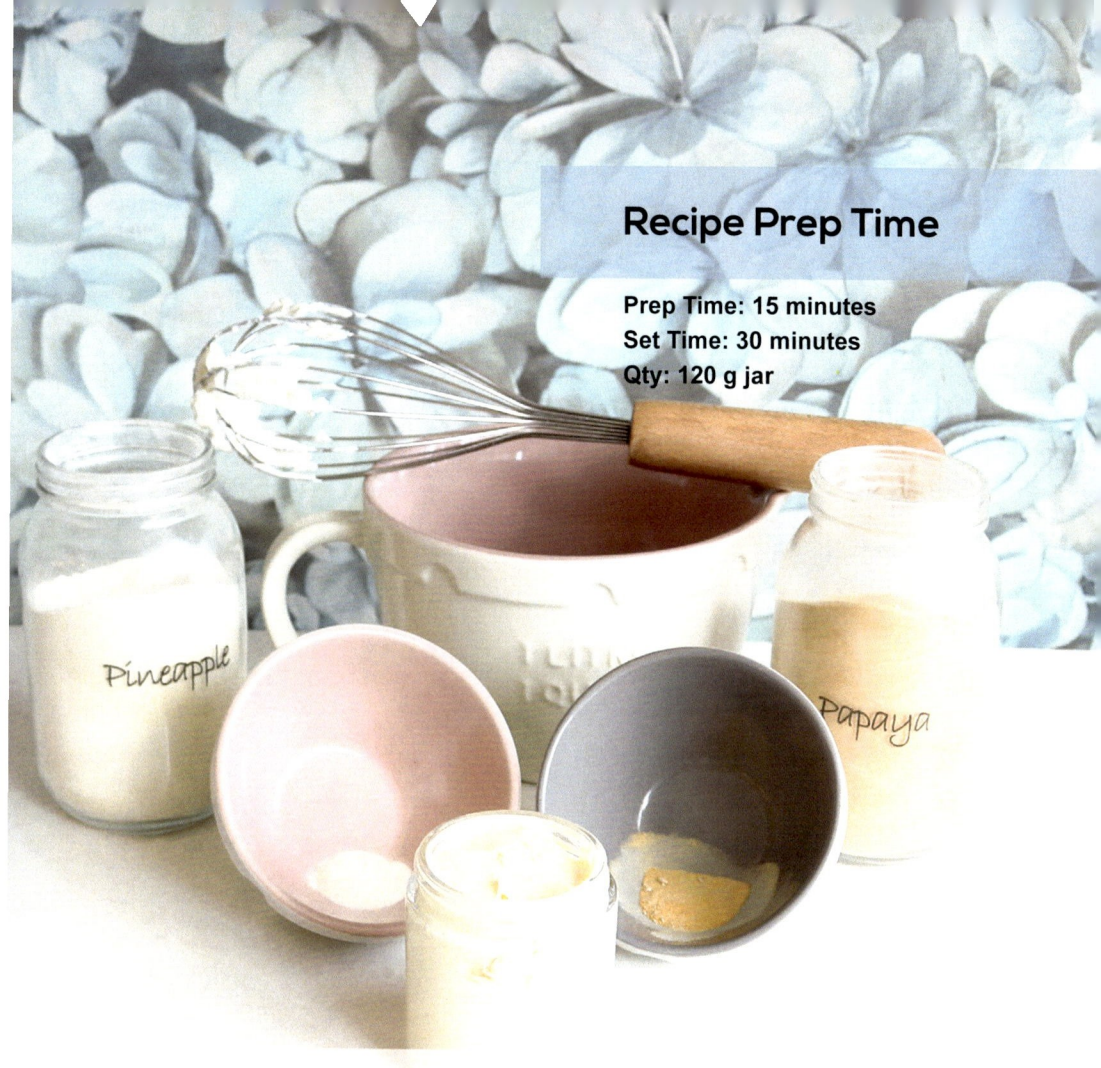

1. In a double boiler, gradually melt the shea butter, cocoa butter and emulsifying wax (pot 1).
2. Once melted, add in the argan and jojoba oil and whisk (pot 1).
3. In a SEPARATE pot (pot 2), heat up the distilled water and add the superfood powders. Whisk.
4. Remove Pot 1 from heat and pour into a clean dry beaker (Beaker 1).
5. Remove Pot 2 from heat and pour into a SEPARATE beaker (Beaker 2).
6. Slowly pour beaker 2 into beaker 1 while whisking (this must be done gradually so take about 2 minutes to complete this step).
7. Leave the mixture in the beaker and out on the counter to cool for about 3 minutes, and then add in the natural preservative, essential oil, sea buckthorn oil and vitamin E. Mix well with a whisk.
8. Pop the beaker into the fridge for about 30 minutes or until semi-solid.
9. You can then fluff it up with an electric hand mixer and transfer the cream to a jar with a spatula.

Retinol A Golden Berry Anti-Aging Face Cream

If smooth and plump skin is what you're after, natural source retinol ingredients like golden berry, rosehip and carrot can do wonders. Retinol (vitamin A) has been shown to stimulate collagen production, smoothing fine lines and wrinkles.

Raw Ingredients:

120 g creamy vegan butter*
20 drops rosehip oil
10 drops carrot oil
1/2 tsp golden berry superfood powder
1/2 tsp carrot superfood powder
10 drops frankincense essential oil (optional)
1 drop vitamin E (MT-50)

Kitchen Tools:

You will need a double boiler, Pyrex or small pot, scale, beaker, whisk, spatula, measuring spoons and a jar.

Recipe Prep Time

Prep Time: 10 minutes
Set Time: 15 minutes
Qty: 120 g jar

Method:

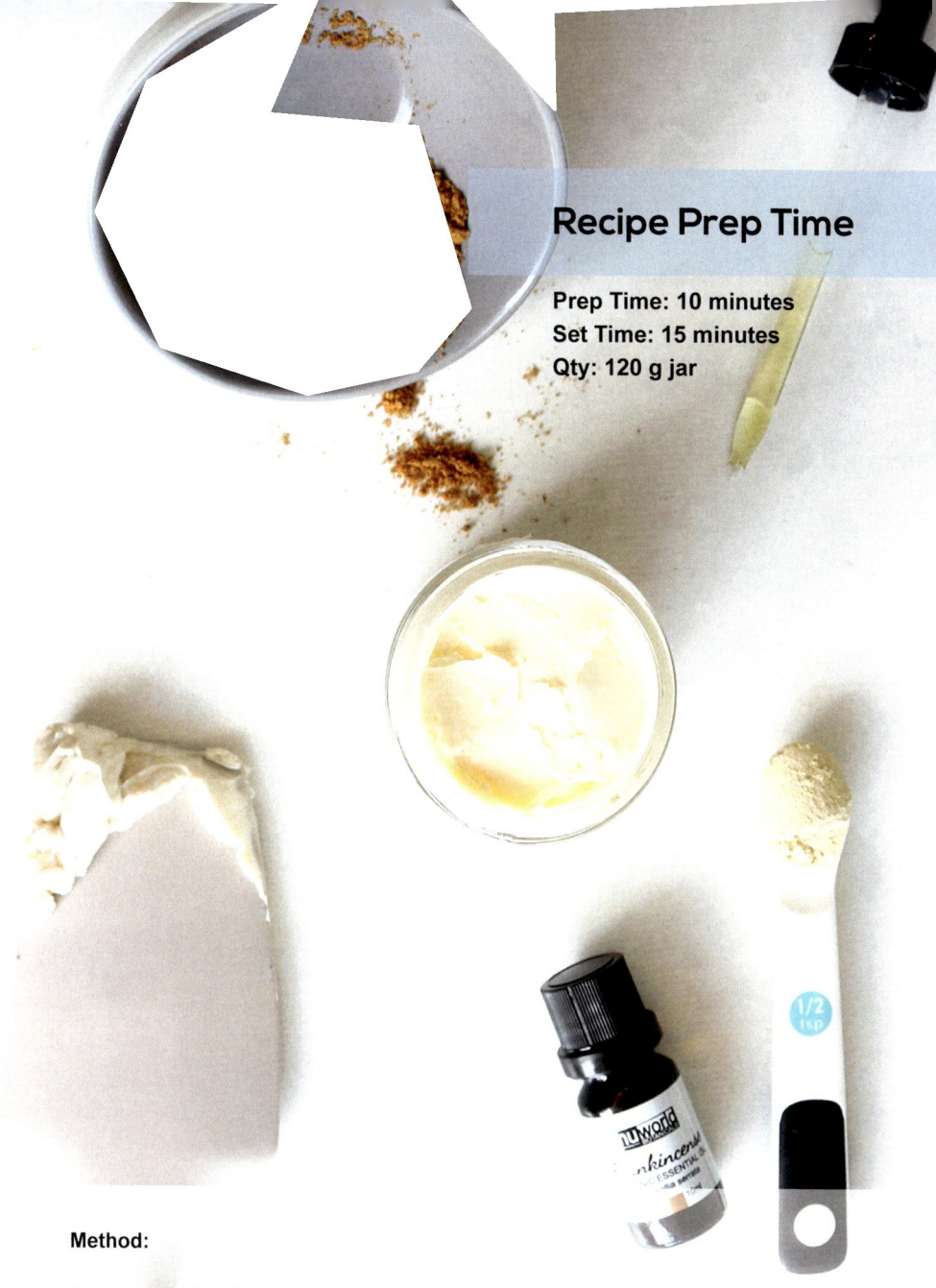

1. In a double boiler, gradually melt down the cream base to a semi-liquid state.
2. Add in the carrier oils.
3. Add in superfood powders and whisk until combined.
4. Transfer the liquid cream into a beaker, add in vitamin E and essential oil and whisk.
5. Pop in fridge for about 15 minutes to set faster or leave out at room temperature to thicken.
6. Transfer mixture into the jar.

Lactic Coconut Collagen Eye Cream

This recipe is loaded with GLA (from Borage oil) and lactic acid to help keep the delicate eye area skin soft and supple. Lactic acid is known to stimulate collagen renewal and can firm your skin. Borage oil restores moisture and helps treat dry skin. It is specifically known for its ability to soothe eczema and dermatitis.

Raw Ingredients:

60 g borage base butter*
5 drops sweet almond oil
5 drops calendula oil
5 drops borage oil
1/4 tsp organic coconut superfood powder
1/4 tsp aloe vera superfood powder
5 drops blue chamomile essential oil
1 drop vitamin E (MT-50)

Kitchen Tools:

You will need a scale, beaker, whisk, spatula, measuring spoons and a jar.

Recipe Prep Time

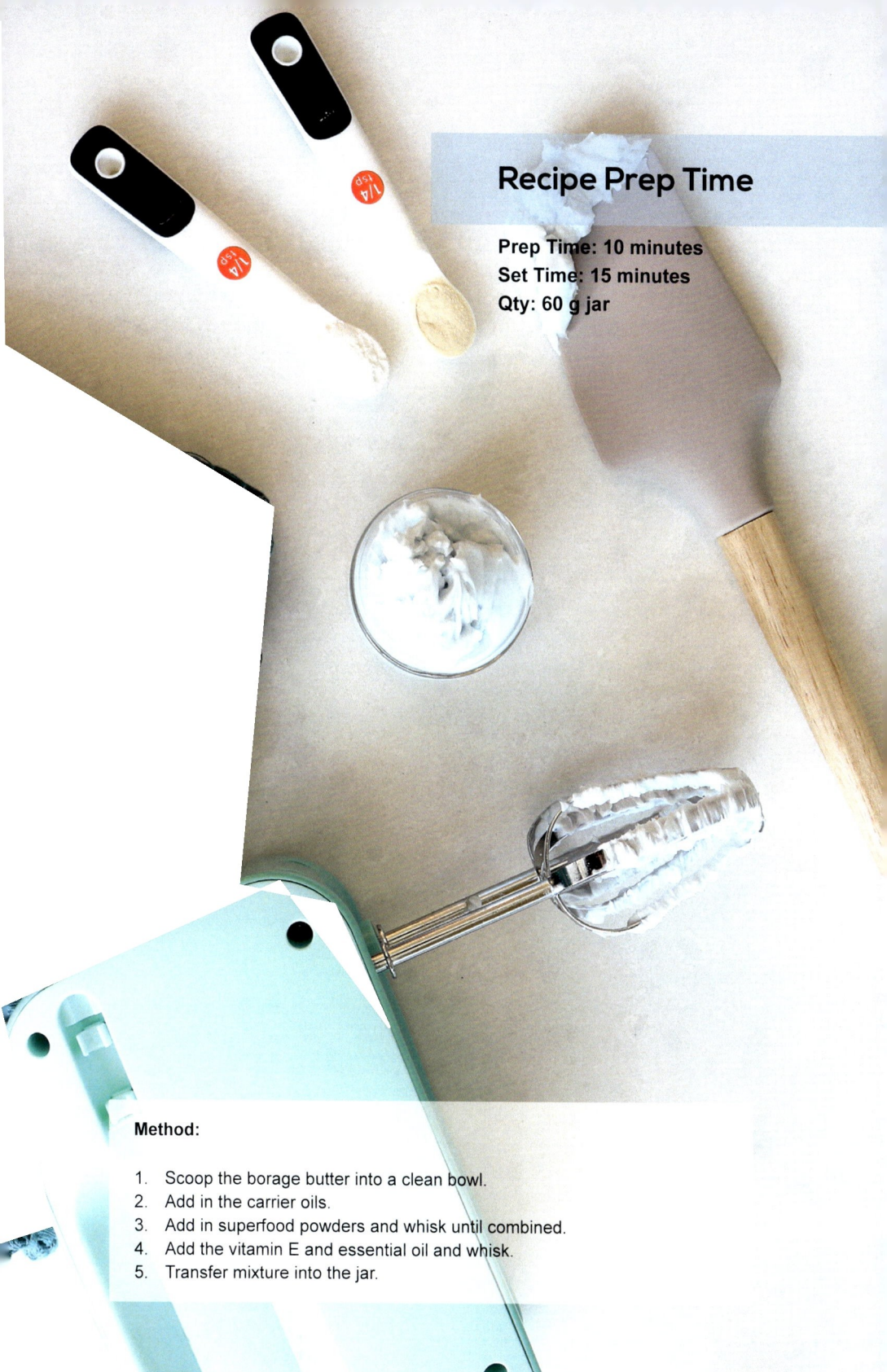

Prep Time: 10 minutes
Set Time: 15 minutes
Qty: 60 g jar

Method:

1. Scoop the borage butter into a clean bowl.
2. Add in the carrier oils.
3. Add in superfood powders and whisk until combined.
4. Add the vitamin E and essential oil and whisk.
5. Transfer mixture into the jar.

HA Banana Face Balm

Boost your skin with natural sources of hyaluronic acid! Banana extract and broccoli oil are abundant sources of magnesium that support hyaluronic-acid production, encouraging supple skin and a bright complexion. Vegan carnauba wax helps thicken this waterless recipe.

Raw Ingredients:

25 g soy butter (non-gmo)
12 g extra virgin coconut oil
10 ml avocado oil
5 ml broccoli oil
1/2 tsp banana superfood powder
2 g carnauba wax
1 drop blue tansy essential oil
1 drop vitamin E (MT-50)

Kitchen Tools:

You will need a double boiler, Pyrex or small pot, scale, beaker, whisk, measuring spoon and a jar.

Recipe

Prep Time: 10 minu...
Set Time: 20 minutes
Qty: 60 g jar

Tip: This product gets its' pretty blue hue from Blue Tansy essential oil.

Method:

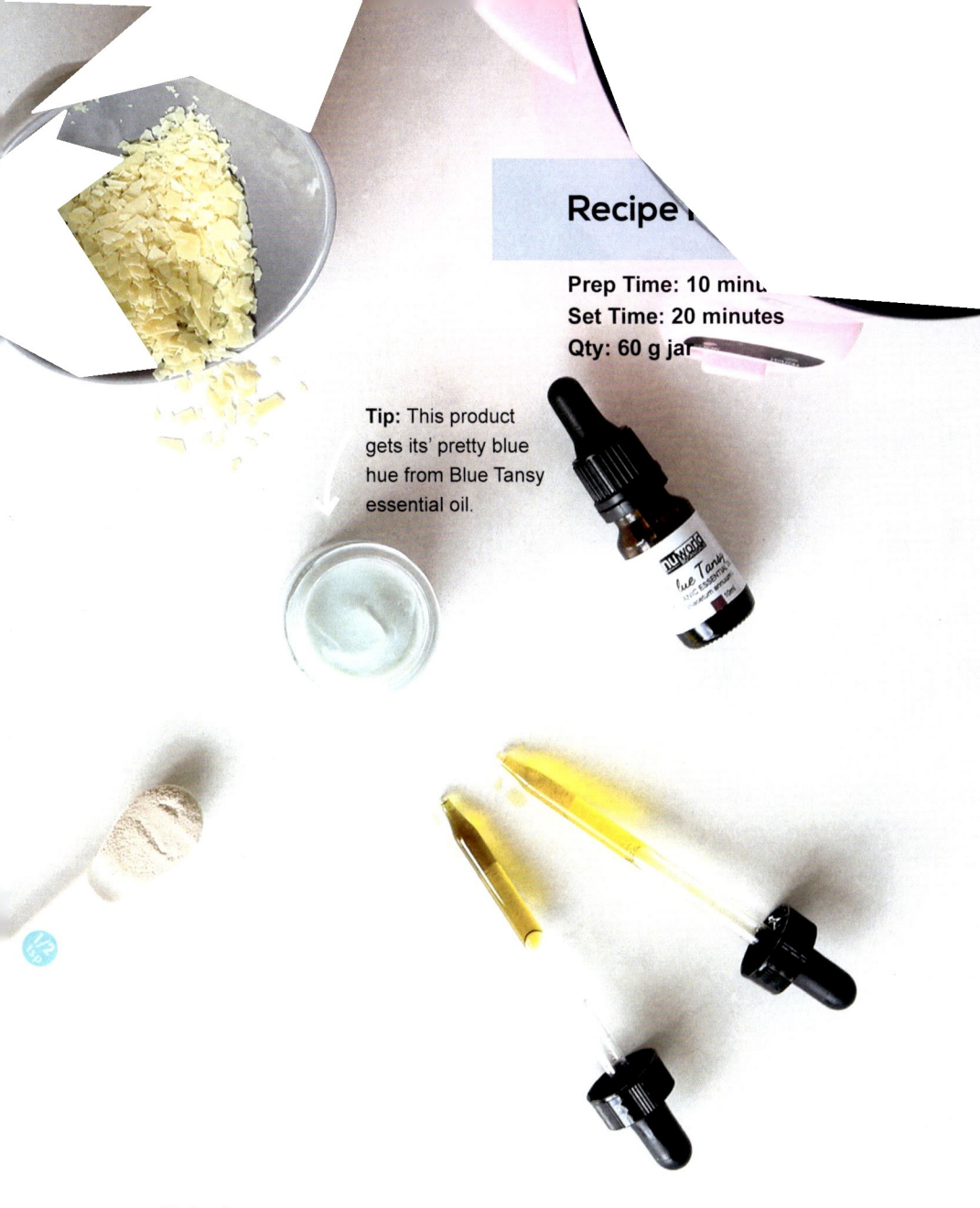

1. In a double boiler, gradually melt down the butter, wax and extra virgin coconut oil.
2. Add in the carrier oils and superfood powders and mix well.
3. Transfer the liquid to the beaker.
4. Add in the vitamin E and essential oil. Mix well.
5. Pour the mixture into the jar.
6. Pop in fridge for 20 minutes to set.

Lactic Acid Apple Sleep Lip Mask

This luxe hydrating lip mask delivers intense moisture and antioxidants while you sleep. Camellia oil contains cell rebuilding nutrients to lock in moisture and vegetable glycerin makes the perfect remedy for dry, chapped lips.

Raw Ingredients:

10 ml vegetable glycerin
1/8 tsp organic coconut superfood powder
1/8 tsp apple cider vinegar superfood powder
9 drops camellia seed oil
3 drops hemp seed oil

Kitchen Tools:

You will need a small bowl, beaker, whisk, measuring spoon and a tube.

Recipe Prep Time

Prep Time: 5 minutes
Set Time: 5 minutes
Qty: 10 ml tube

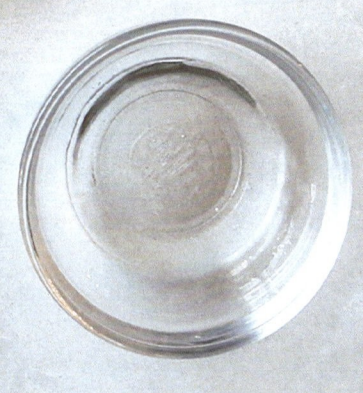

Method:

1. In a small bowl, mix vegetable glycerin and superfood powders.
2. Add in carrier oils and mix.
3. Transfer mixture into a small beaker. Pour into the tube.

Butterfly Pea Collagen Lip Plump + Scrub

Plump and polish with this duo-purpose recipe! Butterfly Pea flower (rich in polyphenols) stimulates the production of collagen, babassu butter delivers superb hydration and tiny beads of Jojoba gently buff and polish your skin.

Raw Ingredients:

10 g shea butter
5 g babassu butter
6 g extra virgin coconut oil
8 ml meadowfoam oil
1 g carnauba wax
1/2 tsp jojoba beads
1/4 tsp butterfly pea superfood powder
1/4 tsp lemon superfood powder
10 drops lemon essential oil

Kitchen Tools:

You will need a double boiler, Pyrex or small pot, scale, beaker, whisk, measuring spoon and a jar.

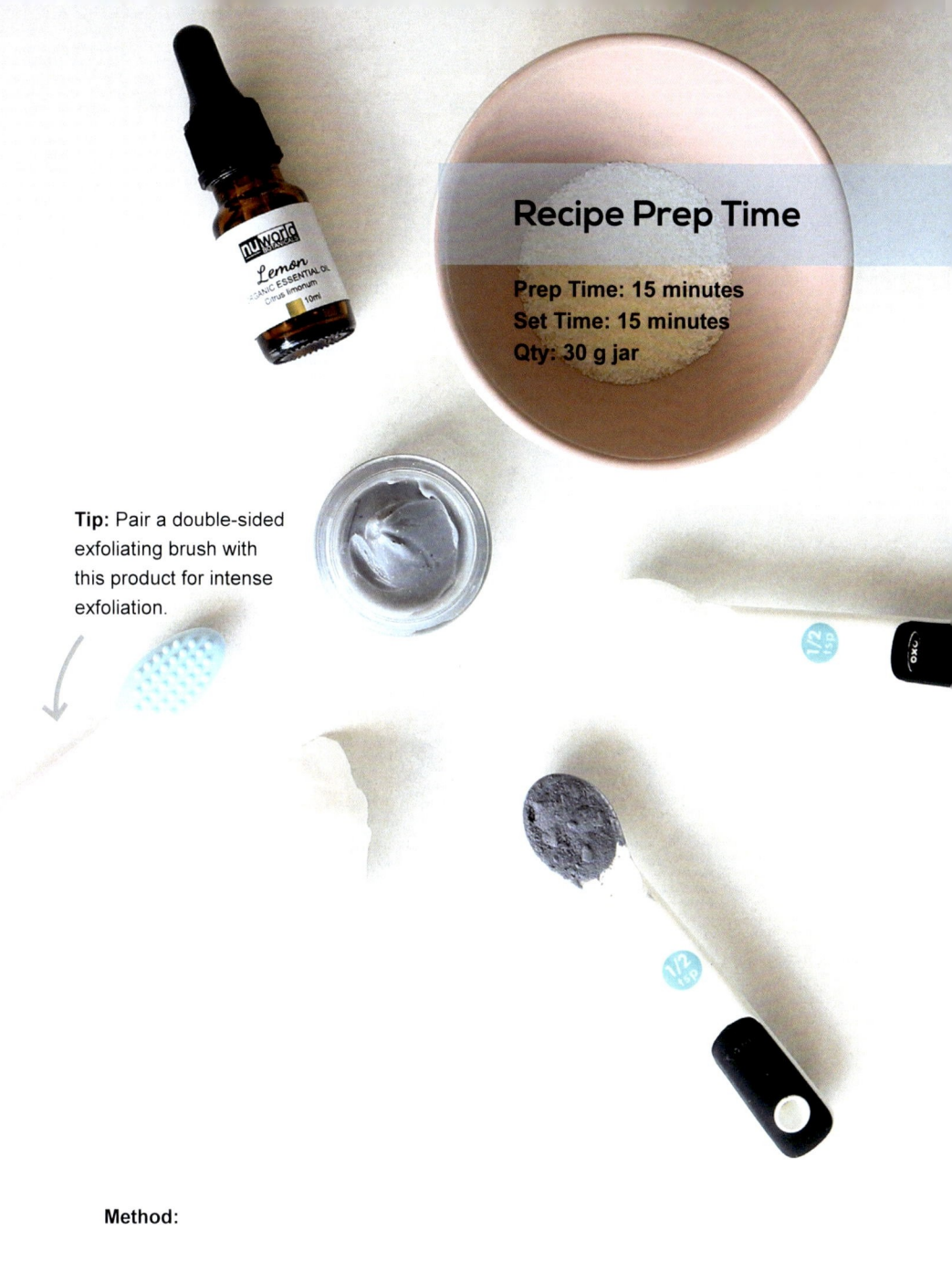

Recipe Prep Time

Prep Time: 15 minutes
Set Time: 15 minutes
Qty: 30 g jar

Tip: Pair a double-sided exfoliating brush with this product for intense exfoliation.

Method:

1. In a double boiler, gently melt down the butters, wax, and coconut oil.
2. Add in carrier oils.
3. Add in superfood powders. Whisk well.
4. Transfer into the beaker and add the jojoba beads and essential oil and mix well.
5. Pour the mixture into a jar (put lid on tightly).
6. Pop in the jar in the fridge for about 15 minutes, to set faster.

Sweet Dreams Aromatherapy Roll-on

Our Sweet Dreams aromatherapy blend is rich with skin-softening vitamin E from jojoba oil and calming essential oils known to promote sleep and relaxation. Roll-on, breathe in and sweet dreams!

Raw Ingredients:

6 ml fractionated coconut oil
3 ml jojoba oil
4 drops lavender essential oil
2 drops chamomile essential oil
2 drops sweet orange essential oil
2 drops geranium essential oil
1 drops patchouli essential oil
1 drop sea buckthorn oil
1 drop vitamin E (MT-50)

Kitchen Tools:

You will need a measuring spoon, funnel and a roll-on bottle.

Recipe Prep Time

Prep Time: 5 minutes
Set Time: 5 minutes
Qty: 10 ml roll-on

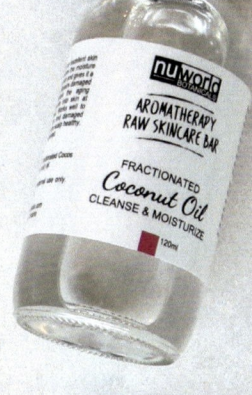

Tip: Roll this sleep elixir on the bottom of your feet just before bed and slip on a pair of cozy socks. Night night!

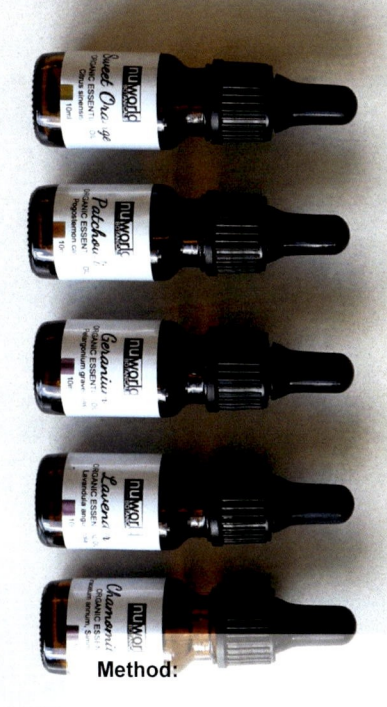

Method:

1. Fill the roll-on bottle with carrier oils (leave room for your essential oils and to pop the roller ball back in).
2. Add in the essential oils.
3. Add in the vitamin E.
4. Pop the roller ball back in and cap.
5. Shake botte and roll-on wellness.

Diy Superfood Bodycare Recipes

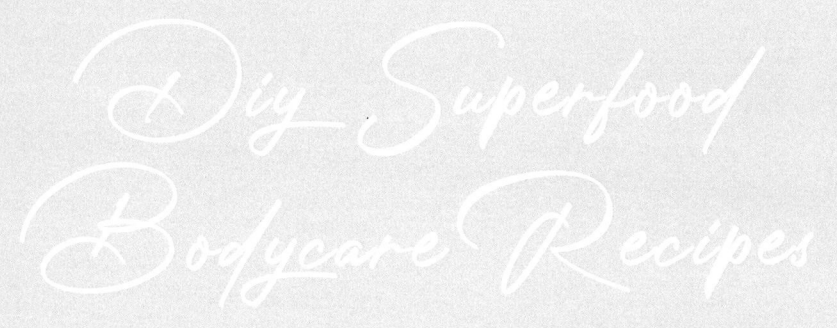

Let's cook, bake and create!

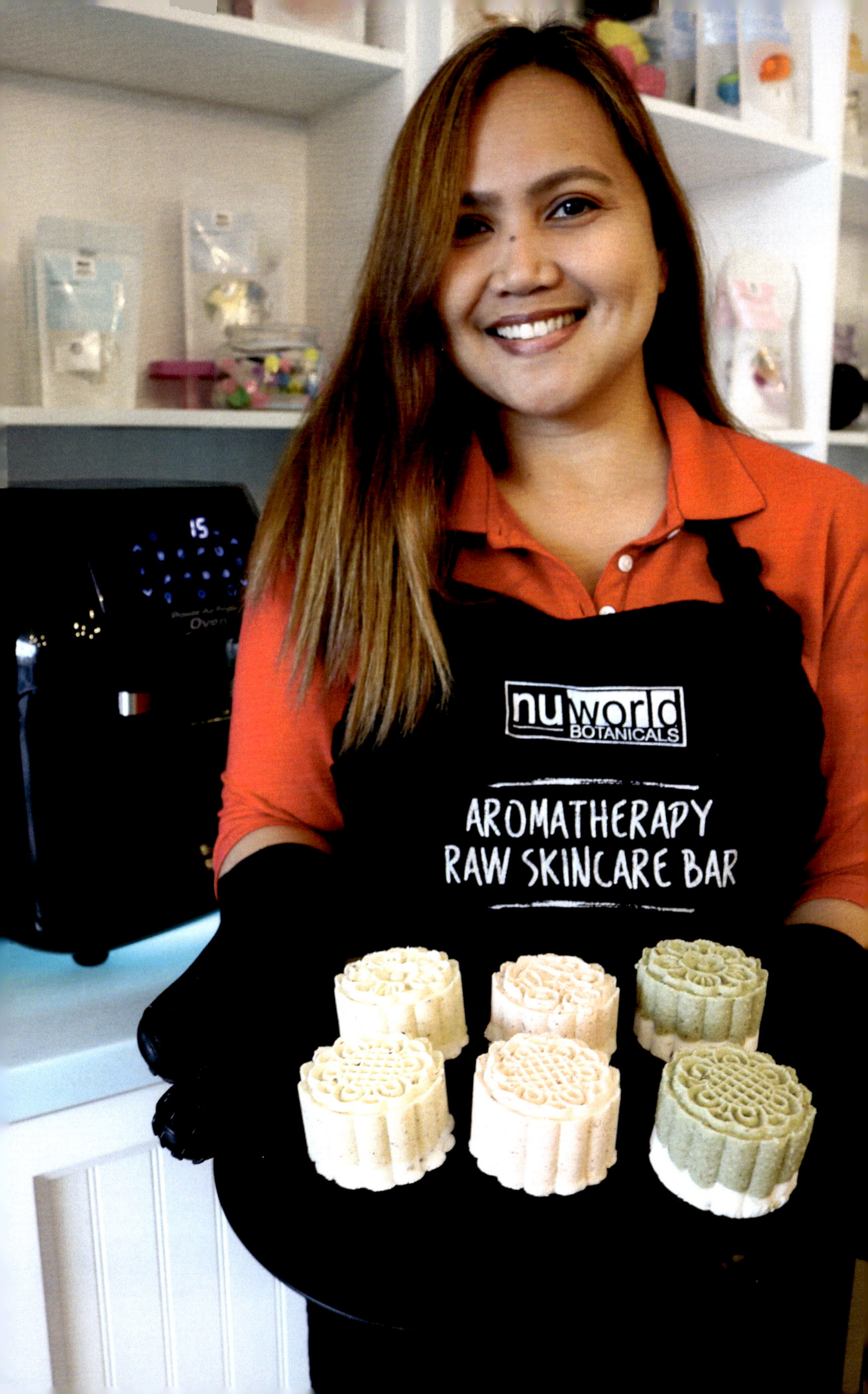
nu world
BOTANICALS
AROMATHERAPY
RAW SKINCARE BAR

Cocoa + Coffee Skin Toning Soapsicle

Rise and shine! Stimulate your senses (and your skin) with the invigorating scent and properties of coffee essential oil. Smells just like a gourmet pot of fresh coffee. This power antioxidant cleansing bar pairs cocoa with coffee to help improve circulation, skin elasticity and skin tone. For topical use only, on body or face.

Raw Ingredients:

120 g shea melt & pour soap base
1/2 tsp cocoa superfood powder
1/8 tsp bamboo leaf superfood powder
1/8 tsp moroccan rhassoul clay
1/8 tsp coffee grinds exfoliant
10 drops coffee essential oil

Kitchen Tools:

You will need a double boiler, Pyrex or small pot, scale, 2 beakers, whisk, spatula, measuring spoon and a silicone mold (popsicle sticks optional).

Recipe Prep Time

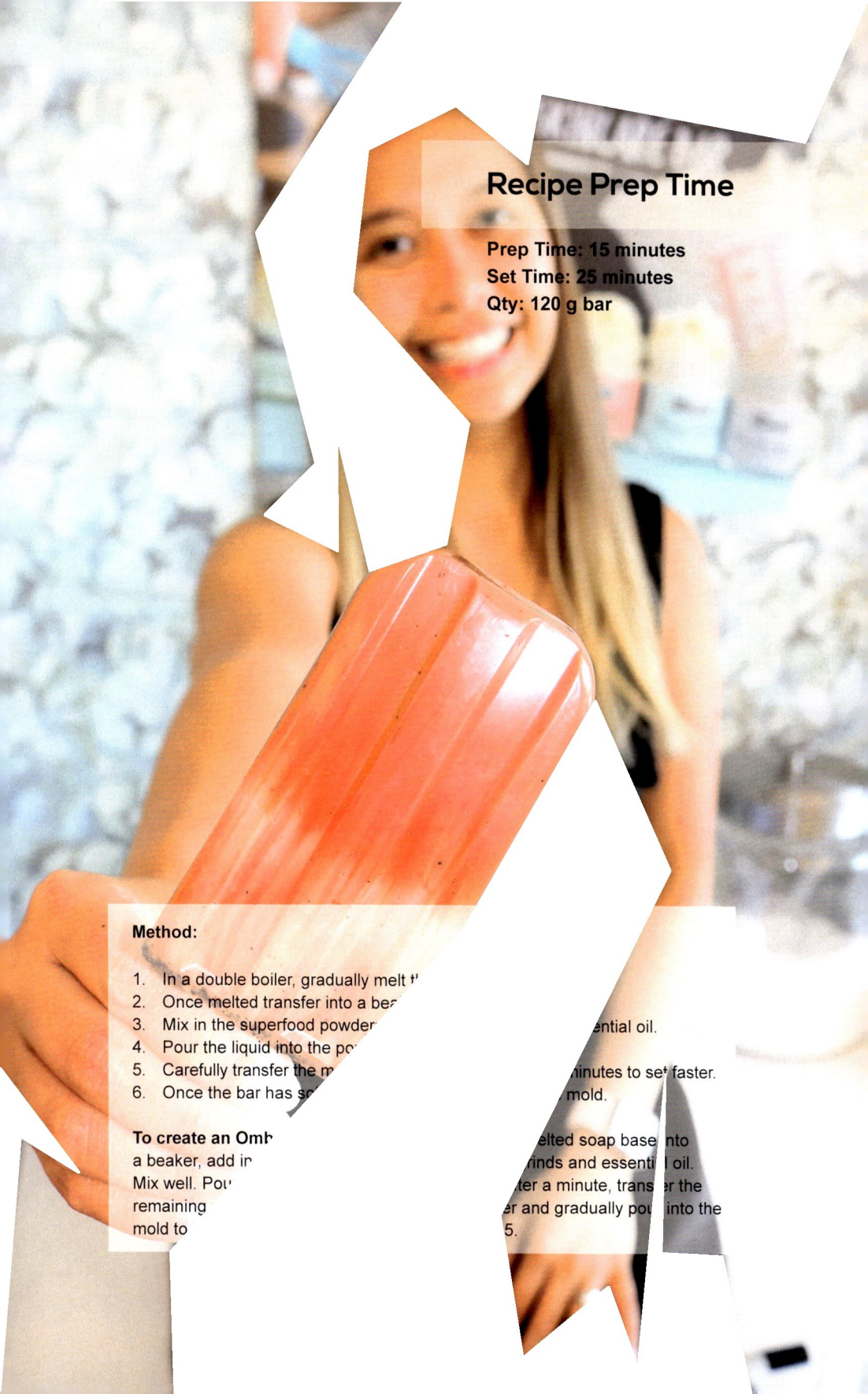

Prep Time: 15 minutes
Set Time: 25 minutes
Qty: 120 g bar

Method:

1. In a double boiler, gradually melt t
2. Once melted transfer into a bea
3. Mix in the superfood powder   ential oil.
4. Pour the liquid into the po
5. Carefully transfer the m   inutes to set faster.
6. Once the bar has s   mold.

To create an Om   elted soap base nto
a beaker, add i   nds and essenti oil.
Mix well. Pou   ter a minute, trans er the
remaining   er and gradually pou into the
mold to   5.

Blue Spirulina Cooling Soapsicle

This Blue Spirulina cleansing bar is a power anti-inflammatory that can help calm down irritated, itchy and stressed skin. Butterfly pea and blue spirulina superfoods are mega-rich in antioxidants that can help relieve inflammation, redness, and even eczema. For topical use only, on face or body.

Raw Ingredients:

90 g aloe melt & pour soap base
1/4 tsp blue spirulina superfood powder
1/8 tsp butterfly pea superfood powder
1/8 tsp of white kaolin clay
3 drops blue tansy essential oil

Kitchen Tools:

You will need a double boiler, Pyrex or small pot, scale, 2 beakers, whisk, spatula, measuring spoon and a silicone mold (popsicle sticks optional).

Recipe Prep Time

Prep Time: 15 minutes
Set Time: 25 minutes
Qty: 90 g bar

Method:

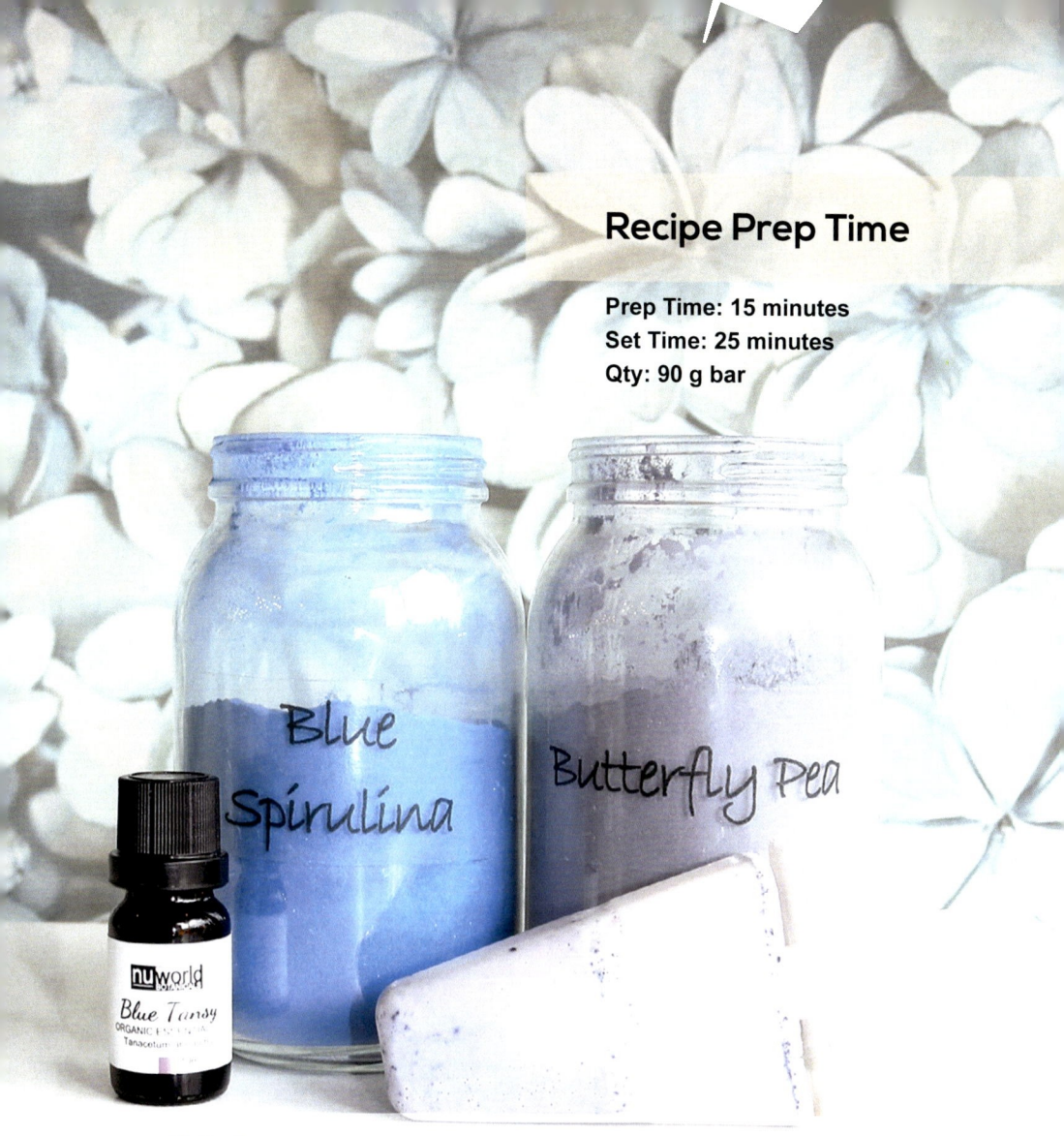

1. In a double boiler, gradually melt the soap base.
2. Once melted transfer into a beaker.
3. Mix in the superfood extracts, clay and essential oil.
4. Pour the liquid into the popsicle mold.
5. Carefully transfer the mold to the fridge for about 25 minutes to set faster.
6. Once the bar has solidified, remove from the popsicle mold.

To create an Ombre bar: At step 2, pour half of the melted soap base into a beaker, add in the superfood powders, clay and essential oil. Mix well. Pour the mixture into the popsicle mold. After a minute, transfer the remaining melted soap base into a separate beaker and gradually pour into the mold to achieve an ombre effect. Proceed to step 5.

Coconut Milk & Honey Waffle Hand Soaps

Cleanse and hydrate your hands with these convenient single-use soaps! Moisturizing coconut milk, antibacterial honey and AHA rich superfruits team up to cleanse, hydrate and soften dry hands.

Raw Ingredients:

100 g mango melt & pour soap base
1/2 tsp organic coconut powder
1/8 tsp guava superfood powder
1/8 tsp mango superfood powder
10 drops of lime essential oil

Kitchen Tools:

You will need a double boiler, Pyrex or small metal pot, scale, 1 beaker, whisk, measuring spoon, spatula, squeeze bottle and waffle silicone mold.

Recipe Prep Time

Prep Time: 15 minutes
Set Time: 25 minutes
Qty: 20 x 5 g mini waffles

Stock your jar with individually sealed soaps wrapped in sustainable bags made from wood pulp!

Method:

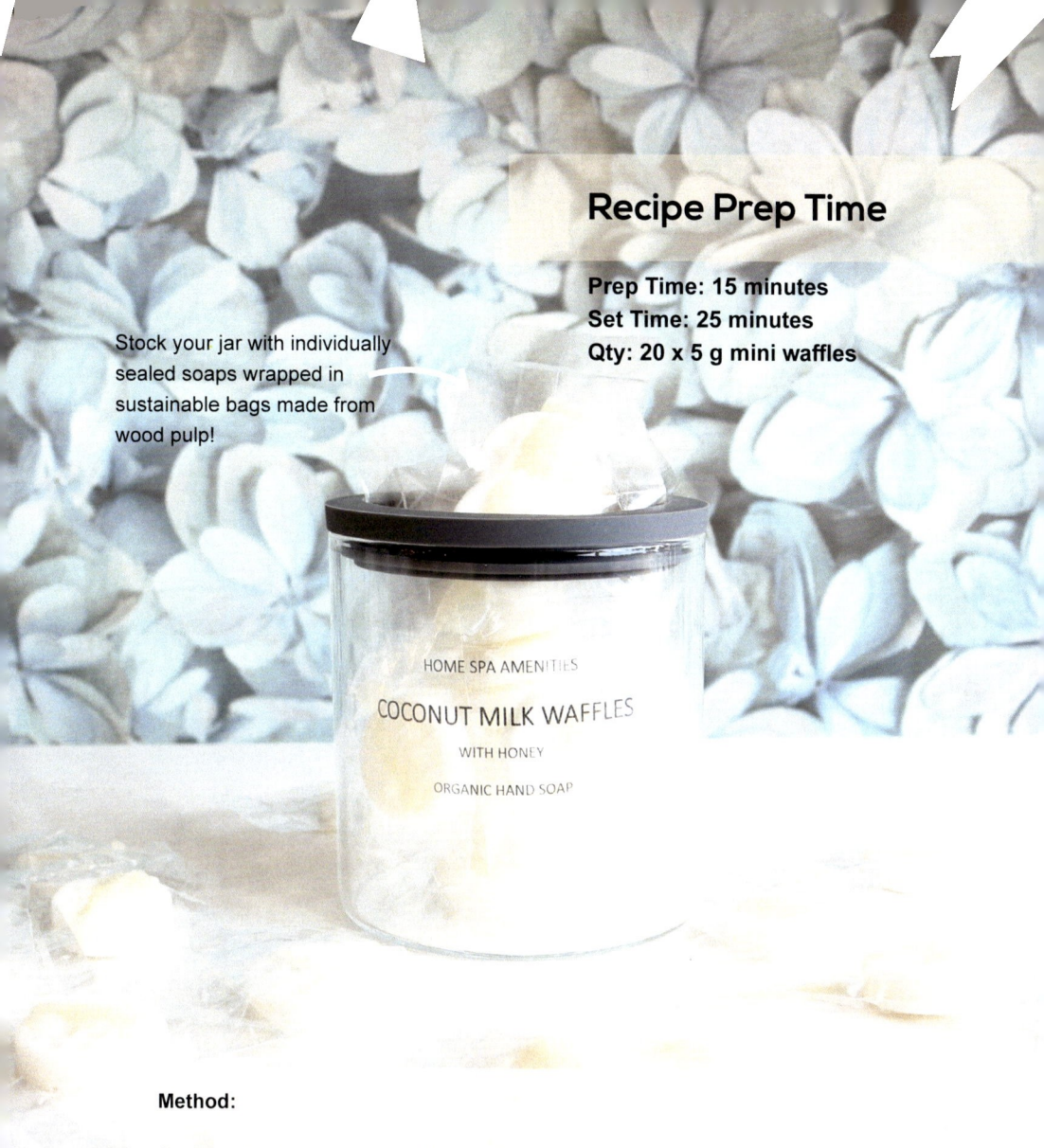

1. In a double boiler, gradually melt the soap base.
2. Once melted transfer into a beaker.
3. Mix in the superfood powders and essential oil. Whisk.
4. Pour the liquid into the waffle mold.
5. Carefully transfer the mold to the fridge for about 25 minutes to set faster.
6. Once the soaps have solidified, remove from molds.

To make honey drizzle icing:

1. In a same pot, melt down 20 g honey soap base.
2. Once melted, transfer it into a squeeze bottle.
3. Working quickly, drizzle overtop the soap.
4. Allow to solidify thoroughly before using.

Power Berry Smoothie Soapsicle

Blueberry, cranberry, strawberry oh my! This cleansing bar contains loads of antioxidants that work on a cellular level to combat skin dullness, dryness, and texture. Together, these berries can help your skin fight inflammation related to acne, psoriasis, eczema, premature aging and support your skin's natural glow. For topical use only, on face or body.

Raw Ingredients:

90 g honey melt & pour soap base
1/8 tsp strawberry superfood powder
1/8 tsp blueberry superfood powder
1/4 tsp cranberry superfood powder
1/8 tsp french pink clay
10 drops lavender essential oil

Kitchen Tools:

You will need a double boiler, Pyrex or small metal pot, scale, 2 beakers, whisk, measuring spoon, spatula, squeeze bottle and silicone mold (popsicle stick optional).

Recipe Prep Time

Prep Time: 15 minutes
Set Time: 25 minutes
Qty: 90 g bar

Method:

1. In a double boiler, gradually melt the soap base.
2. Once melted transfer into a beaker.
3. Mix in the superfood extracts, clay and essential oils.
4. Pour the liquid into the popsicle mold.
5. Carefully transfer the mold to the fridge for about 25 minutes to set faster.
6. Once the bar has solidified, remove from the popsicle mold.

To create a layered bar: At step 2, pour half of the melted soap base into the beaker, add in the superfood powders, clays and 5 drops of essential oil. Mix well. Fill the popsicle molds halfway. Wait until it becomes semi-solid. Transfer the leftover melted soap base to a separate beaker and add in 5 drops of essential oil. Mix well. Pour into mold as a second layer and proceed to step 5.

To make drizzle icing:

1. In a same pot, melt down 20 g shea soap base.
2. Once melted, transfer it into a squeeze bottle.
3. Working quickly, drizzle on top of your soapsicle.
4. Allow bar to solidify thoroughly before using.

Banaba Leaf Magnesium Soapsicle

Banaba (not to be confused with banana) leaf powder is rich in calcium, magnesium and zinc and helps replenish lost minerals. It is also extremely soothing for dry flaky or itchy skin. Add in a dash of green spirulina superfood for cell repair and jojoba beads for mild exfoliation.
For topical use on body or face.

Raw Ingredients:

70 g argan melt & pour soap base
1/8 tsp banaba leaf superfood powder
1/8 tsp green spirulina superfood powder
1/4 tsp green kaolin clay
1/8 tsp jojoba beads (optional)
10 drops of lavender essential oil

Kitchen Tools:

You will need a double boiler, pyrex or small metal pot, scale, beaker, spatula, whisk, measuring spoon and silicone mold (popsicle stick optional).

Recipe Prep Time

Prep Time: 15 minutes
Set Time: 25 minutes
Qty: 70 g bar

Method:

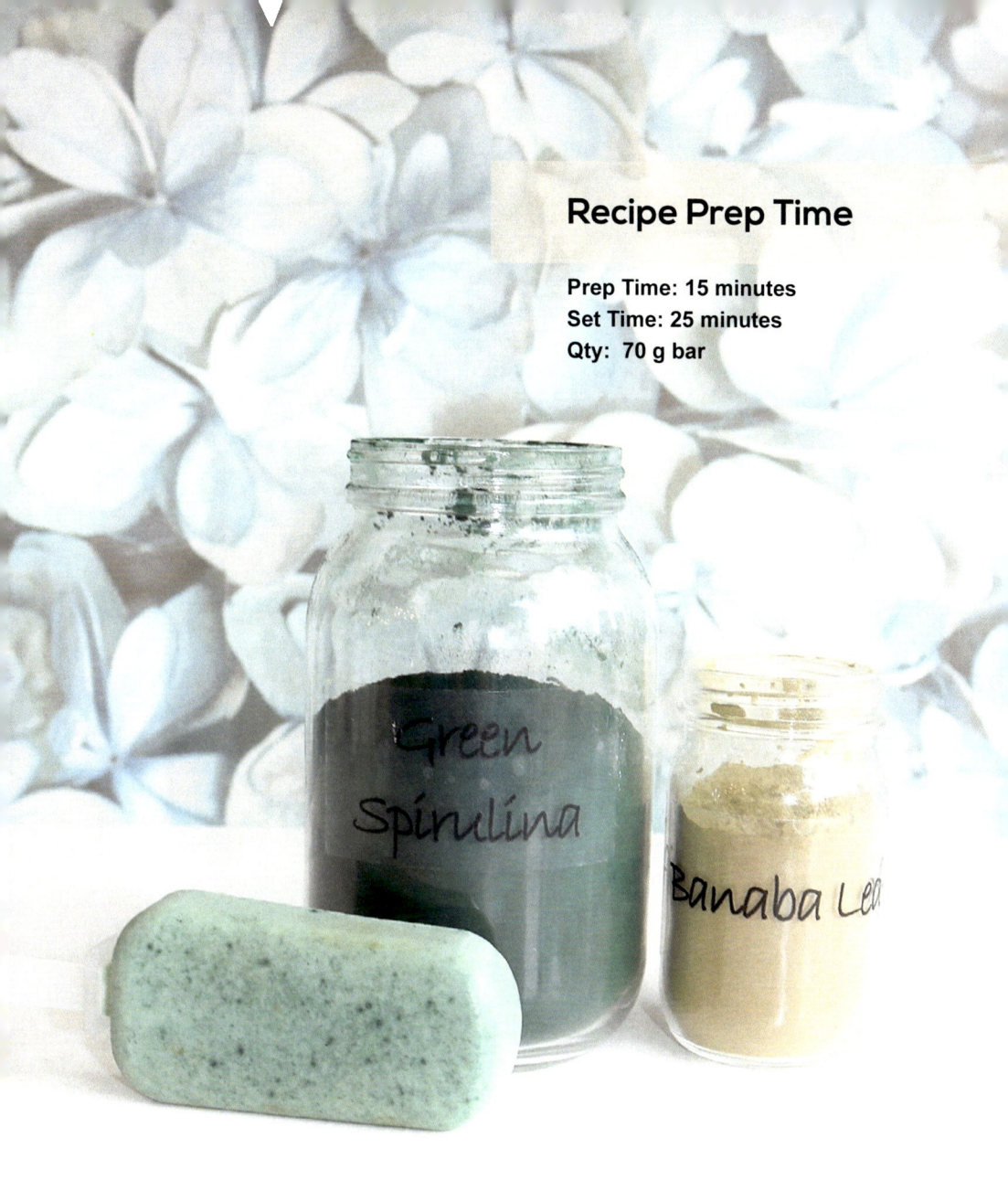

1. In a double boiler, gradually melt the soap base.
2. Once melted transfer into a beaker.
3. Working quickly, mix in the superfood powders, exfoliant, clay and essential oil.
4. Pour the liquid into the popsicle mold.
5. Carefully transfer the mold to the fridge for about 25 minutes to set faster.
6. Once the bar has solidified, remove from the popsicle mold.

Turmeric-Pineapple Glow Soapsicle

Bring out your skin's natural glow! This power bar is chock-full of natural alpha-hydroxy acids (and BHA) that will gently exfoliate the skin to give it that luminous glow. Turmeric can help fight eczema and psoriasis, while sea buckthorn delivers a dash of natural vitamin C. For topical use only, on body or face.

Raw Ingredients:

70 g shea melt & pour soap base
1/4 tsp sea buckthorn superfood powder
1/8 tsp pineapple superfood powder
1/8 tsp turmeric superfood powder
1/8 tsp yellow kaolin clay
1/8 raw loofah exfoliant
2 drops sea buckthorn oil
10 drops sweet orange essential oil

Kitchen Tools:

You will need a double boiler, Pyrex or small metal pot, scale, beaker, whisk, measuring spoon a silicone mold (popsicle sticks optional).

Recipe Prep Time

Prep Time: 15 minutes
Set Time: 25 minutes
Qty: 70 g bar

Method:

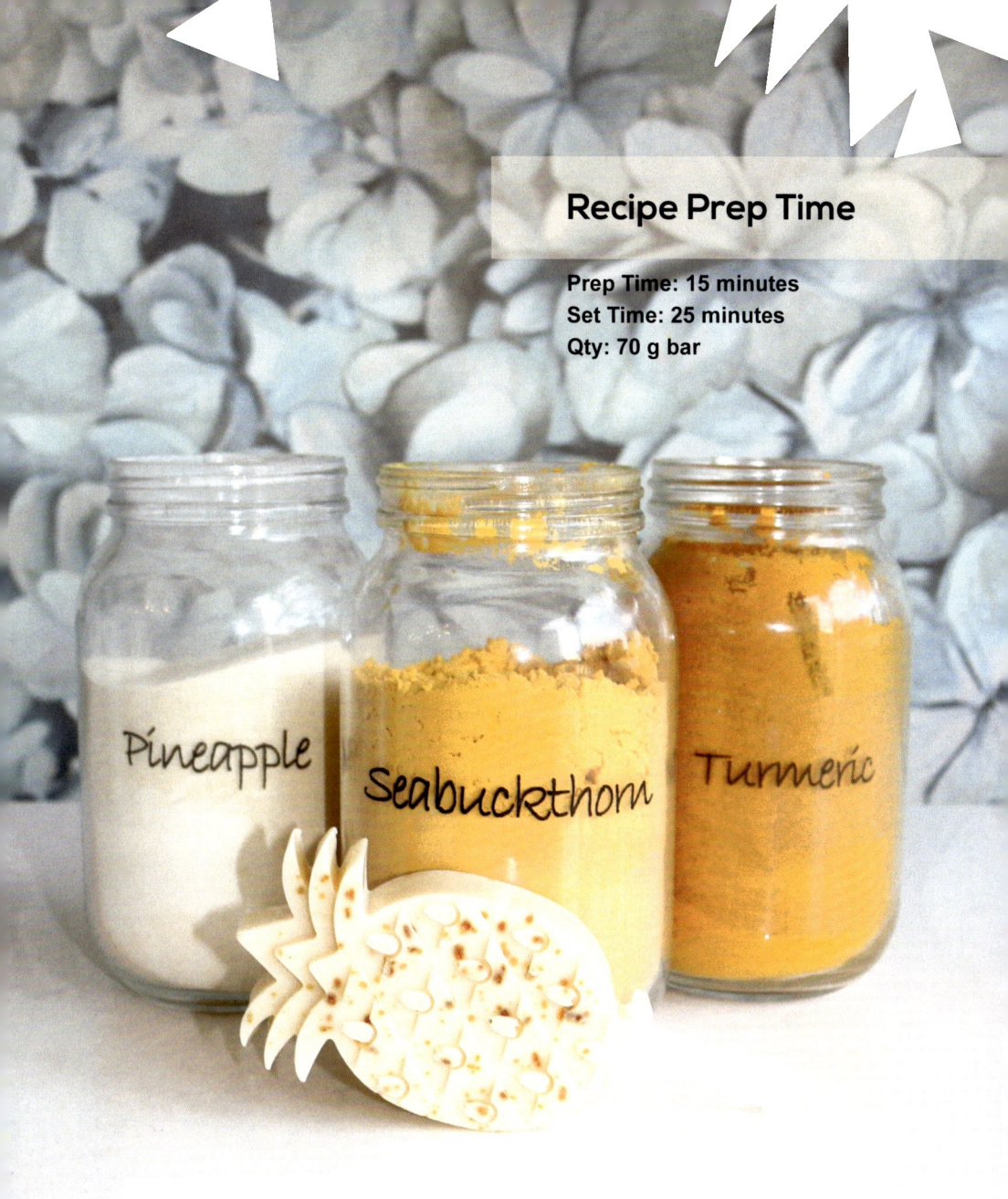

1. In a double boiler, gradually melt the soap base.
2. Once melted transfer into a beaker.
3. Working quickly, mix in the superfood powders, exfoliant, sea buckthorn oil, clay and essential oil.
4. Pour the liquid into the popsicle mold.
5. Carefully transfer the mold to the fridge for about 25 minutes to set faster.
6. Once the bar has solidified remove from the popsicle mold.

Strawberry Vitamin C Soapsicle

Brighten your skin (and your day) with this power superfruit exfoliating cleansing bar. Pink clay gently cleanses and hydrates the skin while superfoods like strawberry and watermelon (rich in AHA and vitamin C) naturally brighten the skin. Add a physical exfoliator like apricot shells to help buff away extra flaky skin. For topical use only, on body or face.

Raw Ingredients:

70 g aloe melt & pour soap base
1/4 tsp strawberry superfood powder
1/4 tsp watermelon superfood powder
1/4 tsp pink kaolin clay
1/4 tsp apricot shells
10 drops rose essential oil

Kitchen Tools:

You will need a double boiler, Pyrex or small pot, scale, beaker, whisk, measuring spoon and silicone mold (popsicle sticks optional).

Recipe Prep Time

Prep Time: 15 minutes
Set Time: 25 minutes
Qty: 70 g bar

Method:

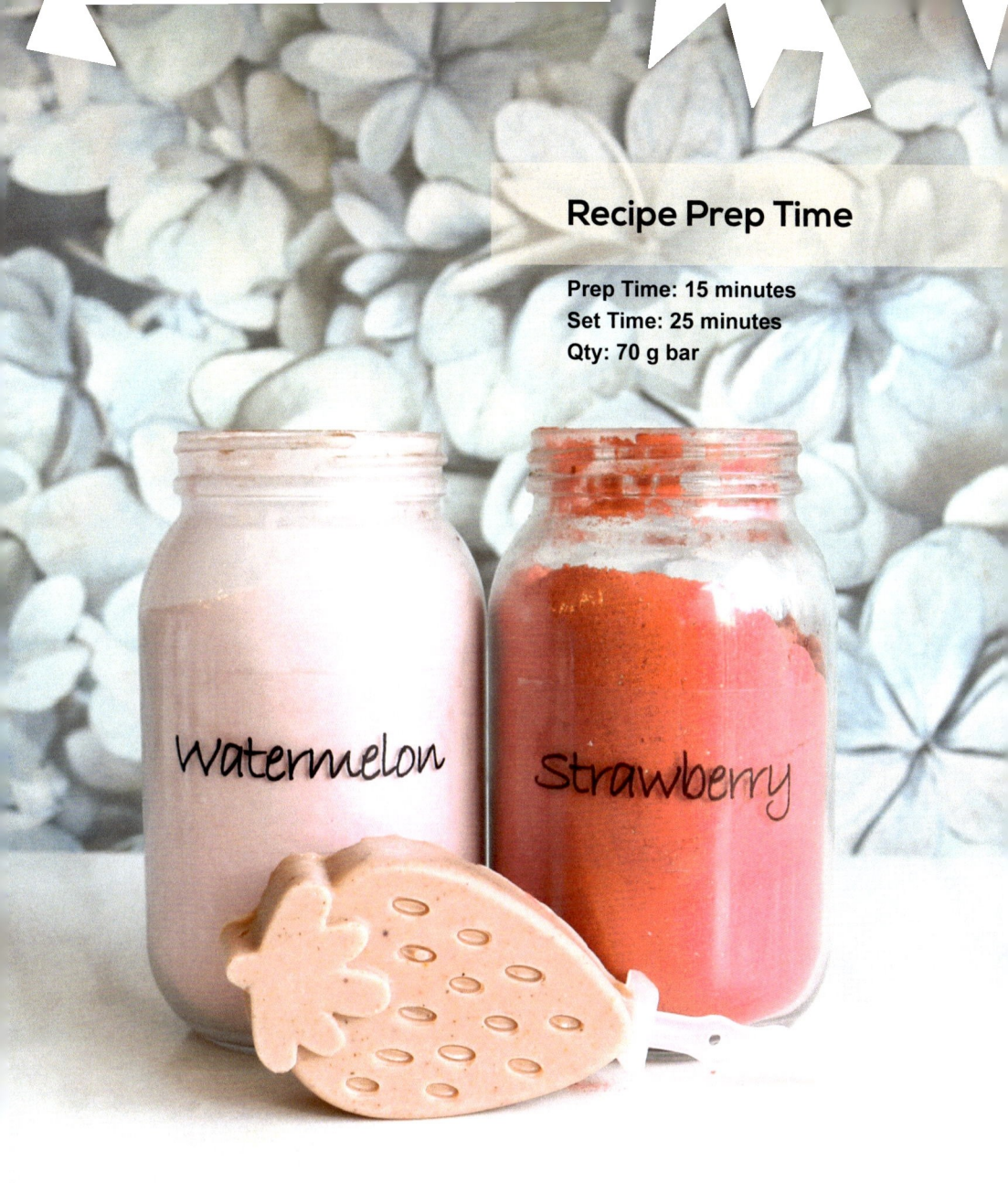

1. In a double boiler, gradually melt the soap base.
2. Once melted transfer into a beaker.
3. Working quickly, mix in the superfood powders, exfoliant, clay and essential oil.
4. Pour the liquid into the popsicle mold.
5. Carefully transfer the mold to the fridge for about 25 minutes to set faster.
6. Once the bar has solidified remove from the popsicle mold.

Superfood Whipped Body Cream

Whip up your favourite superfood body cream from scratch and enjoy the skin-boosting benefits. Blue spirulina can help treat redness and dry itchy skin; mango powder is a rich source of skin-healing antioxidants including vitamin A; hibiscus can help even out skin tone by speeding up cell turnover; and green spirulina fights free radicals.

Raw Ingredients:

20 g shea butter
10 g cocoa butter
20 ml safflower oil
5 ml camellia oil
1 tsp of your favourite superfood powder (ie. blue spirulina, hibiscus, mango, green spirulina)
110 distilled water
15 g emulsifying wax
5 ml natural preservative (Leucidal Liquid Complete)
15 drops lime essential oil
20 drops sweet orange essential oil
2 drops vitamin E (MT-50)

Kitchen Tools:

You will need a double boiler, two metal pots, scale, 2 beakers, measuring spoons, spatula, whisk, an electric mixer and a jar.

Recipe Prep Time

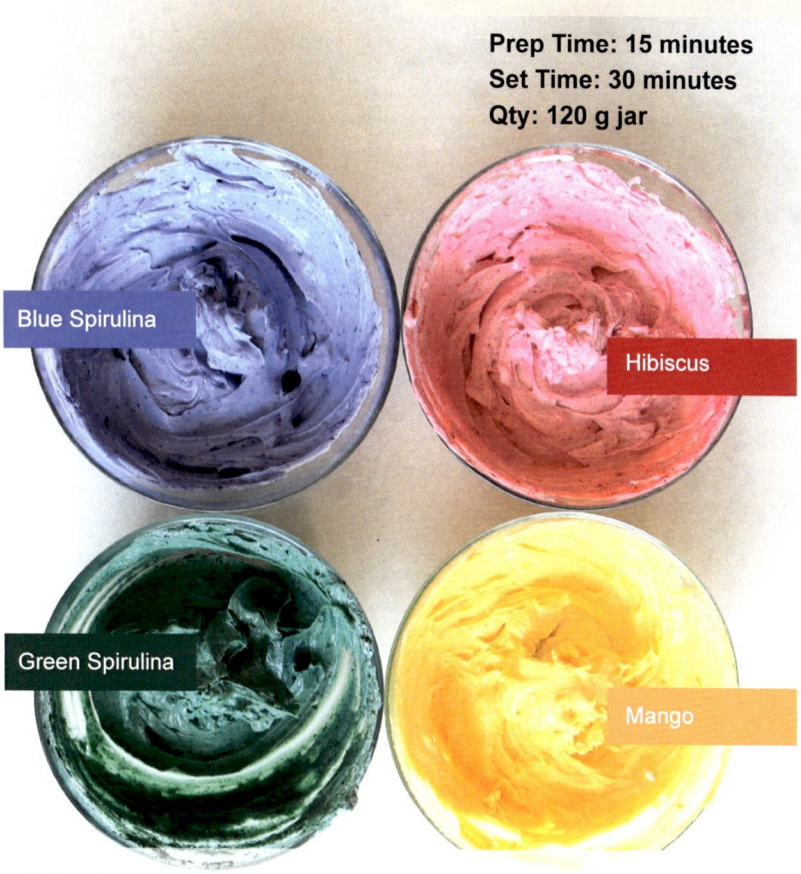

Prep Time: 15 minutes
Set Time: 30 minutes
Qty: 120 g jar

Blue Spirulina

Hibiscus

Green Spirulina

Mango

Method:

1. In a double boiler, gradually melt shea butter and cocoa butter. Add in the emulsifying wax (Pot 1).
2. Once melted, add in the safflower oil and camellia oil (Pot 1).
3. In a SEPARATE pot (Pot 2) heat up the distilled water and add the superfood powder of your choice to the water.
4. Remove Pot 1 from heat and pour into the beaker or Pyrex (beaker 1).
5. Remove Pot 2 from heat and pour into a SEPARATE beaker (beaker 2).
6. Slowly pour Beaker 2 mixture into Beaker 1 while whisking. This must be done slowly. Takes about 2 minutes to complete this step.
7. Leave the beaker out on the counter to cool for about 3 minutes. Add in the natural preservative, vitamin E and essential oils. Mix well.
8. Pop in the fridge for about 30 minutes or until semi-solid.
9. Fluff it up with an electric hand mixer.
10. Transfer the mixture into the jar.

Wolfberry Layered Mineral Bath Soak

Soak up 84-plus minerals with this detox blend of salts and potent superfoods, for radiant skin. Wolfberries are amazing for reducing inflamed and itchy skin, and can also help with acne.

Raw Ingredients:

300 g pink himalayan salt
200 g dead sea mineral salt
20 drops fractionated coconut oil
1/2 tsp wolfberry superfood powder
1/2 tsp cocoa superfood powder
1/2 tsp bamboo leaf superfood powder
10 drops rose essential oil
5 drops geranium essential oil
5 drops rosewood essential oil

Kitchen Tools:

You will need bowls, spatula, dropper, scale, measuring spoon and a jar.

Recipe Prep Time

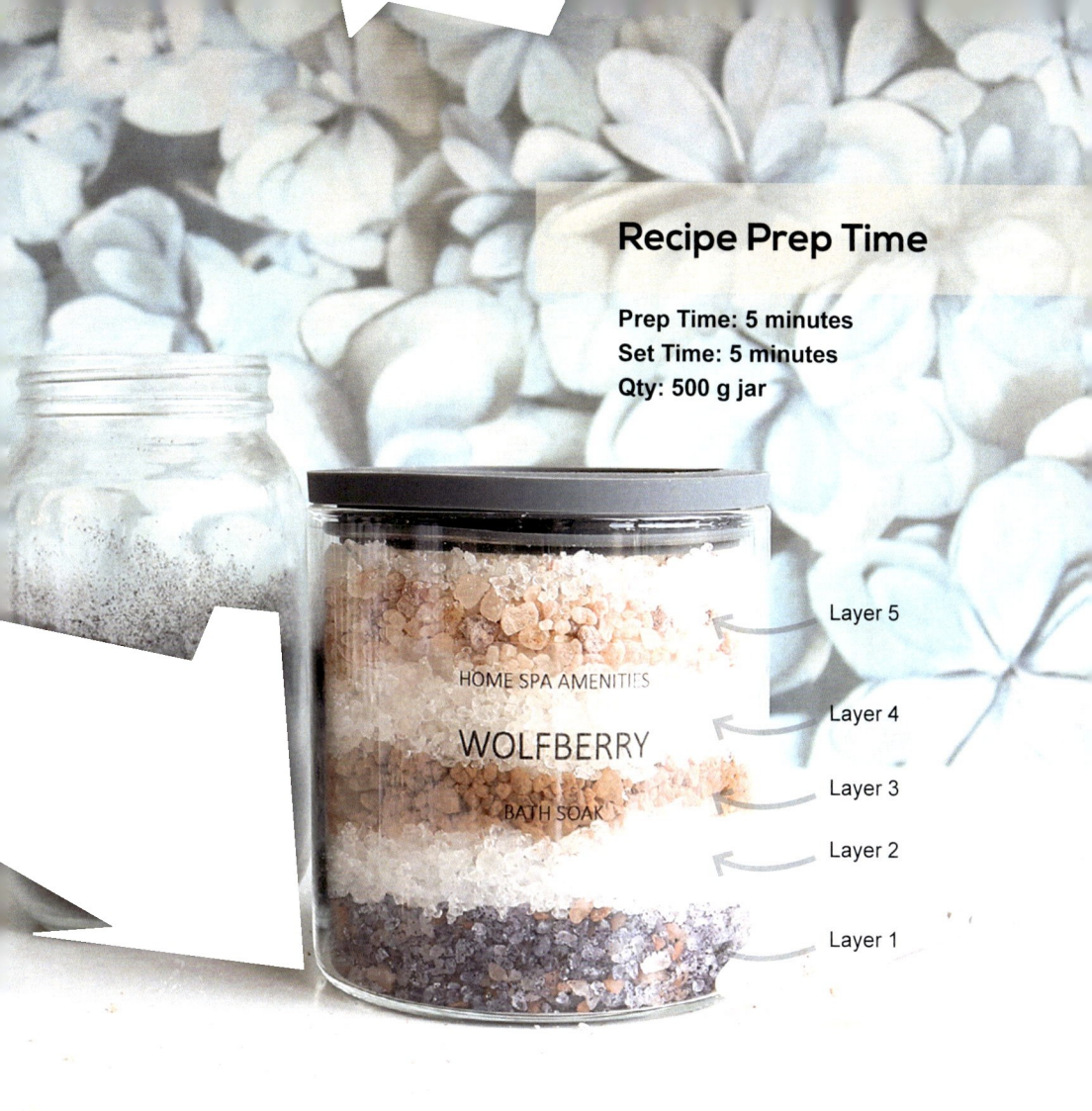

Prep Time: 5 minutes
Set Time: 5 minutes
Qty: 500 g jar

- Layer 5
- Layer 4
- Layer 3
- Layer 2
- Layer 1

Method (Layers):

1. **First Layer:** In a bowl, scoop 100 g of pink himalayan salt. Add 4 drops of carrier oil, 4 drops essential oil and the wolfberry superfood powder. Mix well. Transfer into the jar.
2. **Second Layer:** Scoop in 100 g of dead sea salt into a separate bowl. Add 4 drops of carrier oil, 4 drops essential oil. Mix well. Transfer into the jar.
3. **Third Layer:** In another bowl, weigh 100 g of pink himalayan salt. Add 4 drops of carrier oil, 4 drops essential oil and the cocoa superfood powder. Mix well. Transfer into the jar.
4. **Fourth Layer:** Scoop in 100 g of dead sea salt into a separate bowl. Add 4 drops of carrier oil, 4 drops essential oil. Mix well. Transfer into the jar.
5. **Fifth Layer:** In another bowl, scoop 100 g of pink himalayan salt. Add 4 drops of carrier oil, 4 drops essential oil and the bamboo leaf superfood powder. Mix well. Transfer into the jar.

Pumpkin Mineral Bath Soak

Enjoy a mineral-rich pumpkin sea salt bath! Pumpkin powder is rich in zinc and potassium to help combat redness and reduce skin inflammation. It can also increase the production of collagen, which further improves the tone and elasticity of skin.

Raw Ingredients:

300 g pink himalayan salt
200 g dead sea mineral salt
20 drops fractionated coconut oil
1/2 tsp pumpkin superfood powder
1/2 tsp honey superfood powder
1/2 tsp organic coconut superfood powder
10 drops lemon essential oil
5 drops sweet orange essential oil
5 drops lime essential oil

Kitchen Tools:

You will need a bowl, spatula, dropper, scale, measuring spoon and a jar.

Recipe Prep Time

Prep Time: 5 minutes
Set Time: 5 minutes
Qty: 500 g jar

Method:

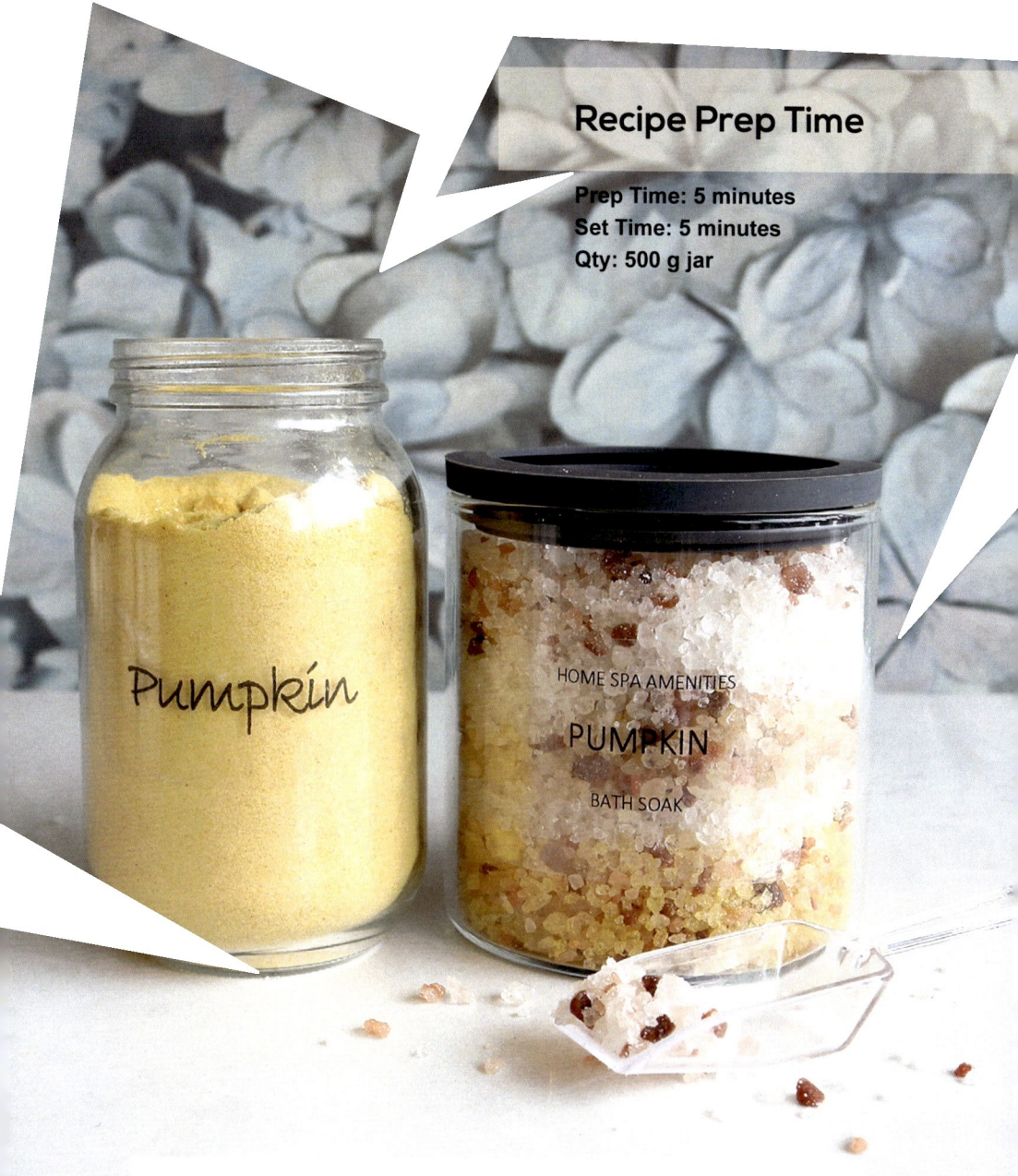

1. Pour pink himalayan salt and dead sea mineral salt into your bowl.
2. Add in the carrier oil (fractionated coconut oil).
3. Add in the essential oils.
4. Add in the superfood powder and mix well.
5. Transfer the mixture into your jar.

Vitamin C Sea Buckthorn Body Oil

Get glowing with one of nature's richest plant sources of vitamin C! Sea buckthorn oil is a brilliant ingredient for aiding in skin repair and regeneration. Naturally brightens the skin and protects skin against free radical damage. Use daily to moisturize, hydrate and protect.

Raw Ingredients:

110 ml apricot kernel oil
5 drops carrot oil
5 drops jojoba oil
10 drops sea buckthorn oil
20 drops essential oil of your choice (optional)

Kitchen Tools:

You will need a funnel and a bottle.

Recipe Prep Time

Prep Time: 5 minutes
Set Time: 5 minutes
Qty: 120 ml bottle

Natural Bronzer: Sea buckthorn oil adds a naturally sun-kissed glow to your skin due to it's high concentration of beta-carotene.

Method:

1. Fill bottle with carrier oils.
2. Add in sea buckthorn oil and essential oils of your choice.
3. Close cap and shake bottle well.

Custom tote and bucket hat are original art-on-fashion, by Elisa Marconi @elisa_art_to_wow.

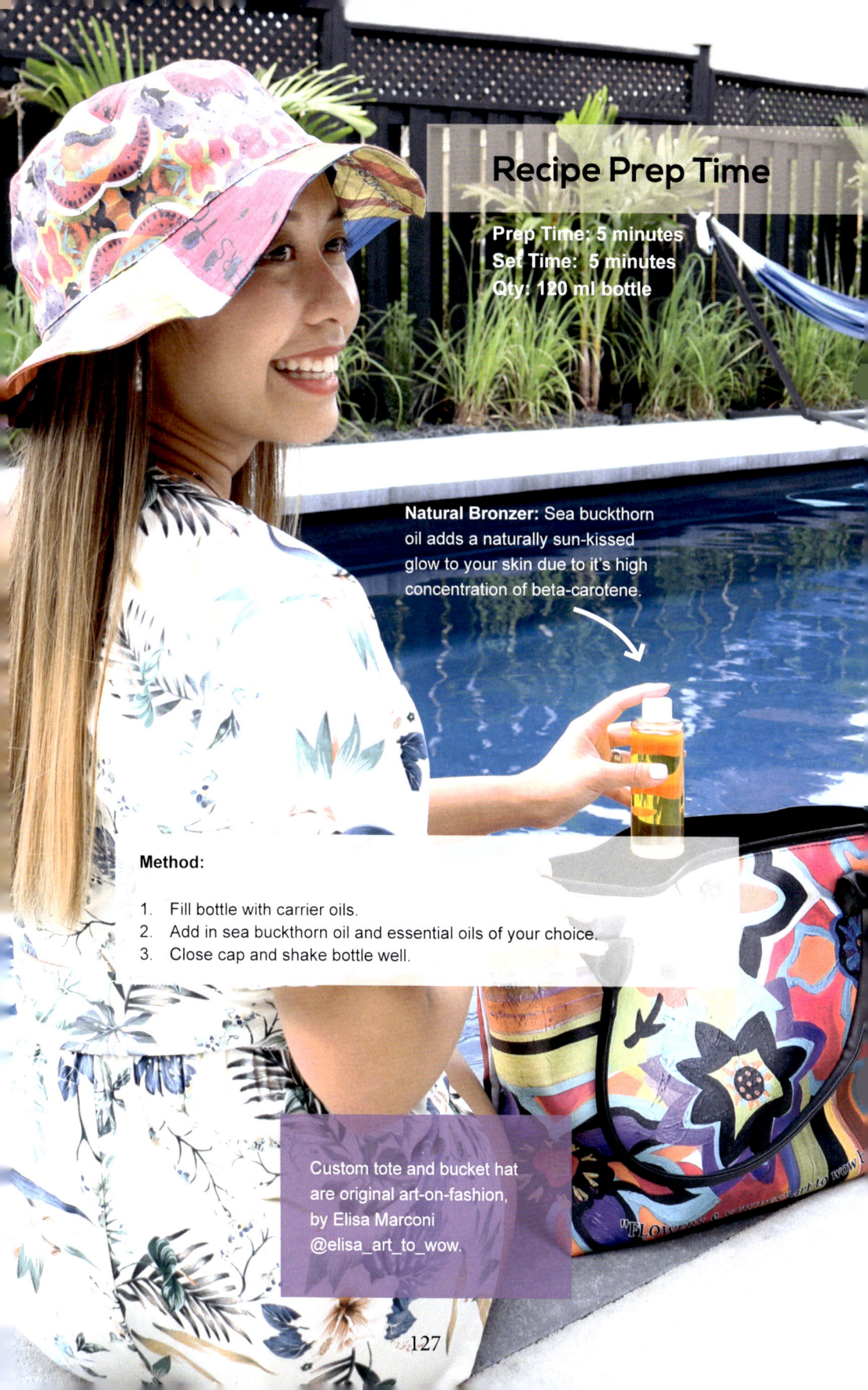

Lemongrass + Loofah Bright Skin Shower Oil

Lemongrass and loofah team up in this vitamin E rich moisturizing shower body oil cleanser. Lemongrass is a power antibacterial and antioxidant. Loofah works its magic to remove dead skin cells to reveal smoother brighter skin.

Raw Ingredients:

115 ml fractionated coconut oil
1 tsp loofah exfoliant
20 drops lemongrass essential oil

Kitchen Tools:

You will need a funnel and a bottle.

Recipe Prep Time

Prep Time: 5 minutes
Set Time: 5 minutes
Qty: 120 ml bottle

Ritual: Use on damp body skin in the shower to naturally cleanse, hydrate and exfoliate.

Method:

1. Using a funnel, add loofah into the bottle.
2. Fill bottle with the fractionated coconut carrier oil.
3. Add in the lemongrass essential oil.
4. Close cap and shake bottle well.

Blue Coconut Milk Layered Bath Fizz

For your bath time routine, try this gourmet bath bomb in a jar with cleansing blue clay, superfood powders and natural fizz. Tie a ribbon around the jar and it makes for a pretty gifting item.

Raw Ingredients:

50 g sodium bicarbonate
20 g citric acid
20 g arrowroot powder
20 g dead sea mineral salt (ultra fine)
10 g pink Himalayan salt
1/2 tsp serbian blue clay
1/2 tsp coconut superfood powder
1/2 tsp butterfly pea superfood powder
15 ml sweet almond oil
10 drops spearmint essential oil

Kitchen Tools:

You will need three bowls, a measuring spoon, whisk, scale, gloves and a jar.

Recipe Prep Time

Prep Time: 10 minutes
Set Time: 10 minutes
Qty: 120 g jar

Layer 3
Layer 2
Layer 1

Method:
1. In a large bowl, combine the sodium bicarbonate, citric acid, arrowroot powder, pink himalayan salt, dead sea ultra fine clay and superfood extract.
2. Wearing gloves, mix well with your hands making sure the mixture is clump-free.
3. Add in the carrier oil (sweet almond) and essential oil and whisk.
4. Transfer mixture into the jar.

To make coloured layers:
1. In a large bowl combined the sodium bicarbonate, citric acid, coconut powder, arrowroot powder and both salts. Mix wearing gloves.
2. Add in the carrier oil (sweet almond) and essential oil. Whisk.
3. Transfer about 1/2 of the mixture into two separate bowls. Add the butterfly pea powder in one bowl and add the blue clay in the other bowl. Mix.
4. Now you make three different coloured layers: white (layer 1), light blue (layer 2) and purple (layer 3).

Avocado Waterless Superfood Balm

Our famous everything balm recipe will nourish and hydrate your face, lips and body. Perfect for extremely dry skin and eczema. Great for sensitive skin types.

Raw Ingredients:

25 g raw shea butter
12 g extra virgin organic coconut oil
15 ml avocado oil
2 g carnauba wax
1 drop vitamin E (MT-50)

Kitchen Tools:

You will need a double boiler, small pot, scale, whisk, spatula, measuring spoons, beaker and a jar.

Recipe Prep Time

Prep Time: 10 minutes
Set Time: 20 minutes
Qty: 60 g jar

Tip: You can use an electric hand mixer once the balm has solidified, to get this fluffy texture.

Method:
1. In a double boiler, gradually melt down the butter, wax and extra virgin organic coconut oil.
2. Add in the carrier oil. Whisk.
3. Transfer mixture into a beaker.
4. Add in the vitamin E and mix well.
5. Then pour liquid into a jar (put the cap on tightly).
6. Pop in the fridge for 20 minutes to set.

Baked Potato Aromatherapy Shower Melts

Enjoy a spa-like ritual every morning and night in your shower. Use invigorating essential oils for morning melts and calming essential oils for evening shower melts.

Raw Ingredients:

110 g sodium bicarbonate
55 g citric acid
55 g arrowroot powder
40 g dead sea ultra fine salt
1/2 tsp white kaolin clay
1 tsp sweet potato superfood powder
10 ml witch hazel
1.25 natural preservative (Leucidal Liquid Complete)
20 drops grapefruit essential oil
20 drops lime essential oil

Kitchen Tools:

You will need a bowl, measuring spoons, spatula, scale, gloves, spray bottle, air fryer (optional) and molds.

Recipe Prep Time

Prep Time: 20 minutes
Set Time: 30 minutes
Qty: 10 x 10 g mini melts

Tip: Amp up the colour by doubling up on your superfood powder measurements, or mix and match colour tones (see our Superfood Colour Guide).

Method:

1. In a large bowl combine: sodium bicarbonate, citric acid, arrowroot powder, dead sea ultra fine salt, clay and sweet potato superfood powder
2. Wearing gloves, mix well with your hands making sure the mixture is a clump free.
3. Add in the essential oils, natural preservative and mix together.
4. Spray mixture with witch hazel; continue to spray until mixture holds together without crumbling (until it mimics wet sand).
5. Pack mixture into mini melt mold.
6. Pop in the fridge for 5 minutes.
7. Quick Dry: Set the air fryer to 170° F (dehydration setting) and bake for 10 minutes. Ready to use.
8. Alternatively, let the mold sit out at room temperature overnight. Remove from molds and enjoy.

Press n' Bake Mineral Superfood Bath Bombs

Press and bake your way to mineral rich goodness! Soak up 84-plus minerals and antioxidants, and enjoy the natural superfood coloured fizz. Now that's a bath bomb with benefits.

Raw Ingredients:

110 g sodium bicarbonate
55 g citric acid
55 g arrowroot powder
1/2 tsp clay (ie. green clay, pink clay, yellow clay)
40 g dead sea mineral salt
20 g pink himalayan salt
1/2 tsp superfood powder extract (ie. matcha, pomegranate, mango)
15 ml safflower oil
10 ml witch hazel (spray)
1.25 natural preservative
20 drops spearmint essential oil
20 drops eucalyptus essential oil

Kitchen Tools:

You will need 2 bowls, measuring spoons, scale, gloves, air fryer (optional), spray bottle and a bath bomb press.

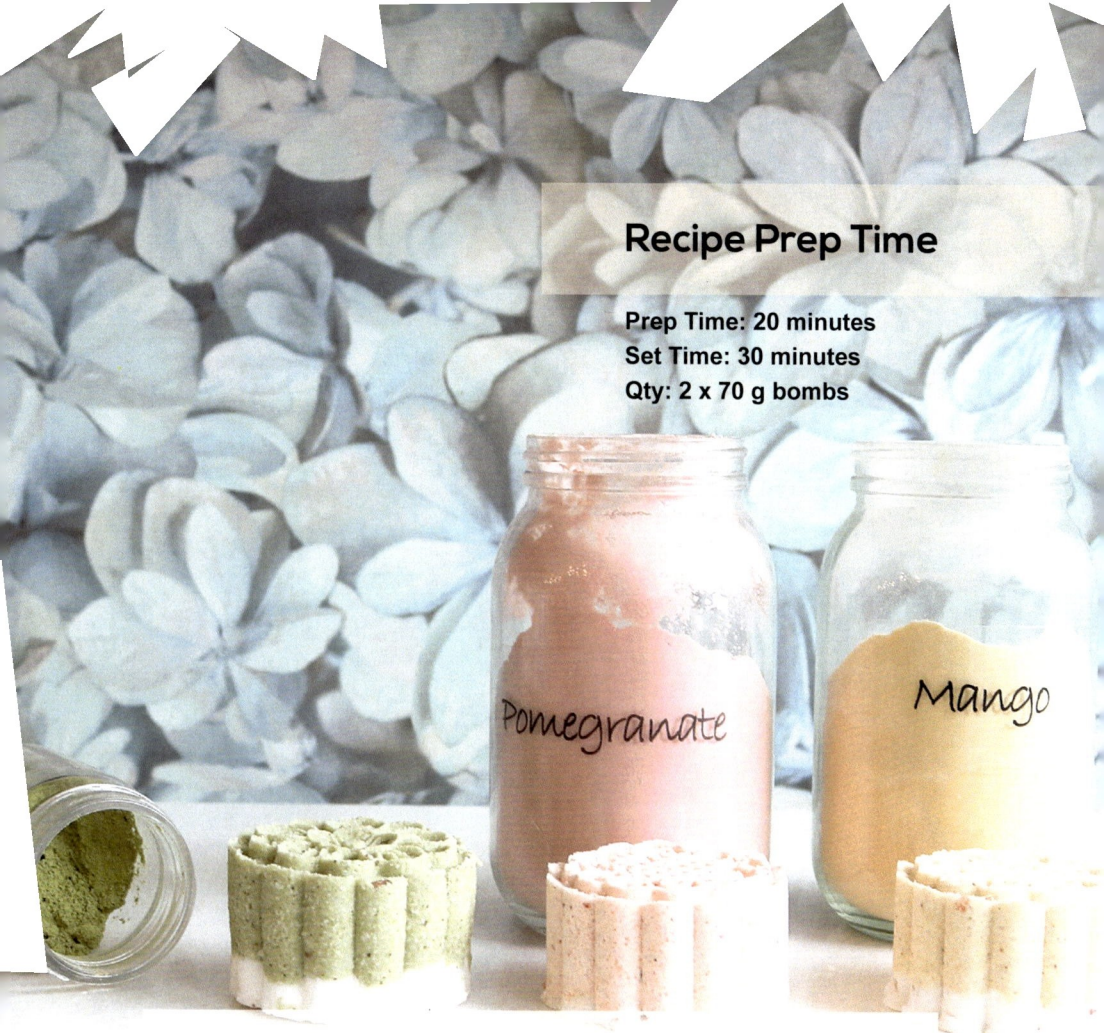

Recipe Prep Time

Prep Time: 20 minutes
Set Time: 30 minutes
Qty: 2 x 70 g bombs

Method:

1. In the first bowl, combine sodium bicarbonate, citric acid, arrowroot powder, dead sea salt and pink himalayan.
2. Wearing gloves, mix well with your hands making sure the mixture is a clump free.
3. Add in safflower oil, natural preservative and the essential oils and mix together.
4. Spray mixture with witch hazel; continue to spray until mixture holds together without crumbling (until it mimics wet sand).
5. In a second bowl, scoop half of the mixture; add the clay and superfood extract powder. Mix well.
6. Take some mixture from the second bowl and pack your bath bomb presser halfway with the mixture.
7. Take some mixture from the first bowl and pack the rest of your presser.
8. Place the presser on a flat surface or tray and release the bath bomb.
9. Quick Dry: Set the air fryer to 170° F (dehydration setting) and let it bake for 10 minutes. It's ready to use.
10. Alternatively, let the bath bombs sit out at room temperature overnight and enjoy the next day.

Raspberry Layered Salt-Balm Body Scrub

Layers and layers of skin-nourishing goodness await! This dessert-like scrub is hand-packed with layers of raw ingredients and superfoods to exfoliate, hydrate and replenish lost minerals. Use in the shower or tub on damp body skin and soak up pure heaven.

Raw Ingredients:

500 g dead sea mineral salt
30 ml fractionated coconut oil
40 g extra virgin coconut oil
1/4 tsp hibiscus superfood powder
1/4 tsp raspberry superfood powder
1/4 tsp cranberry superfood powder
15 drops sandalwood essential oil
5 drops ylang ylang essential oil

Kitchen Tools:

You will need a bowl, spatula, dropper, scale, measuring spoon, scooper and a jar.

Recipe Prep Time

Prep Time: 5 minutes
Set Time: 5 minutes
Qty: 500 g jar

Layers (top to bottom):
- Hibiscus
- Base Mix
- Cranberry
- Base Mix
- Raspberry

Method:

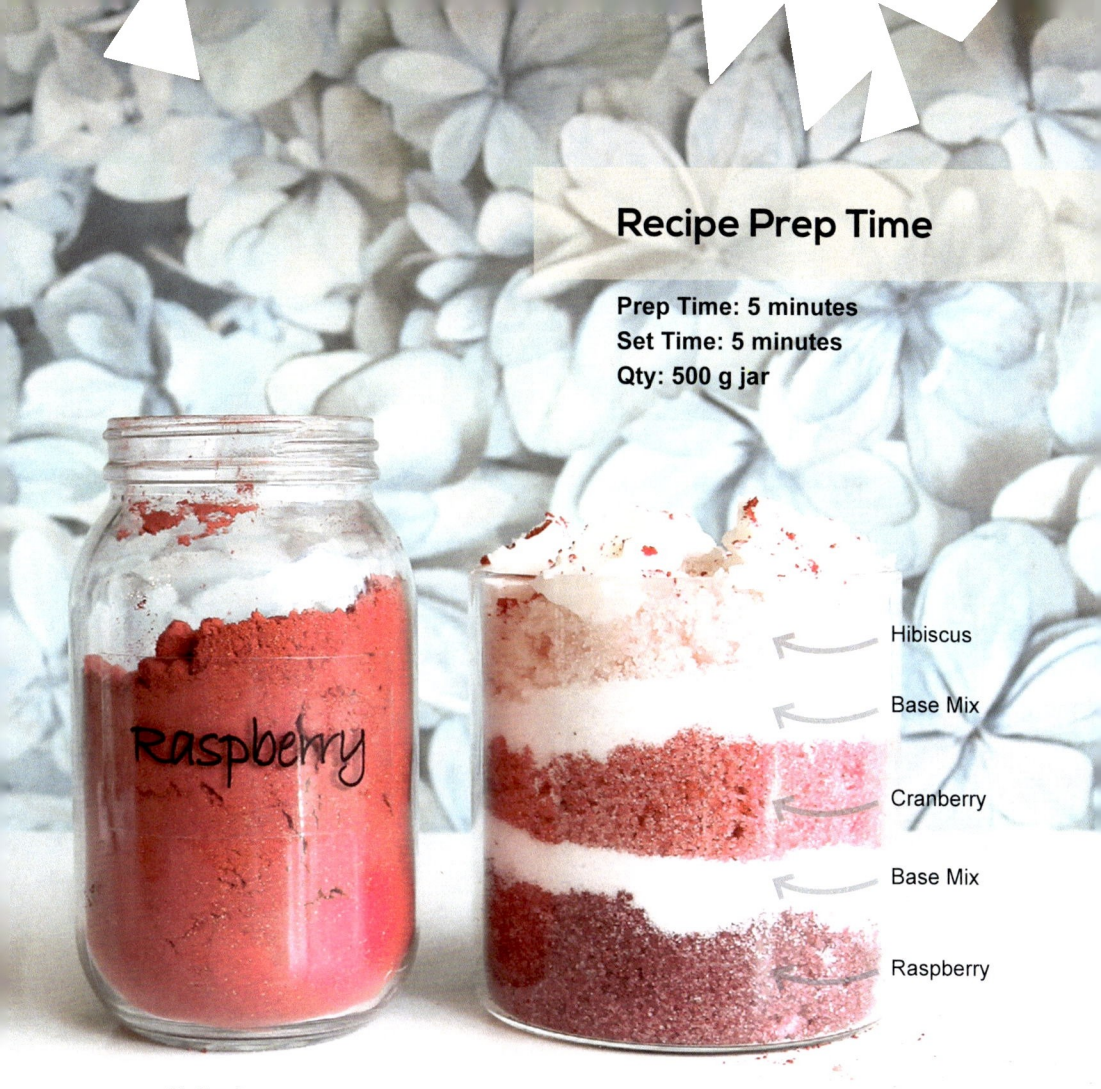

1. Pour dead sea salt into your bowl and add in the extra virgin coconut oil.
2. "Wet" the salt-balm with the carrier oil (fractionated coconut).
3. Add in the essential oils.
4. Add in the superfood extract powders.
5. Mix all of the ingredients together and hand pack in a jar.

To make layers:

1. At step 4 (before you add the colourful superfood powders), divide the 'base mixture' into 4 separate bowls as follows:
2. Bowl 1: 200 g the base mixture (white).
3. Bowl 2: 100 g; add the hibiscus superfood powder and mix well.
4. Bowl 3: 100 g; add the raspberry powder and mix well.
5. Bowl 4: 100 g; add the cranberry superfood extract and mix well.
6. Fill and layer your jar as you wish.

Diy Raw Haircare Recipes

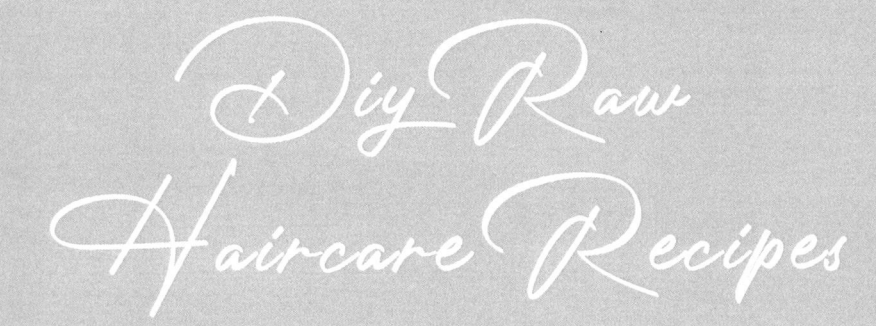

Condition, treat and repair.

MASK

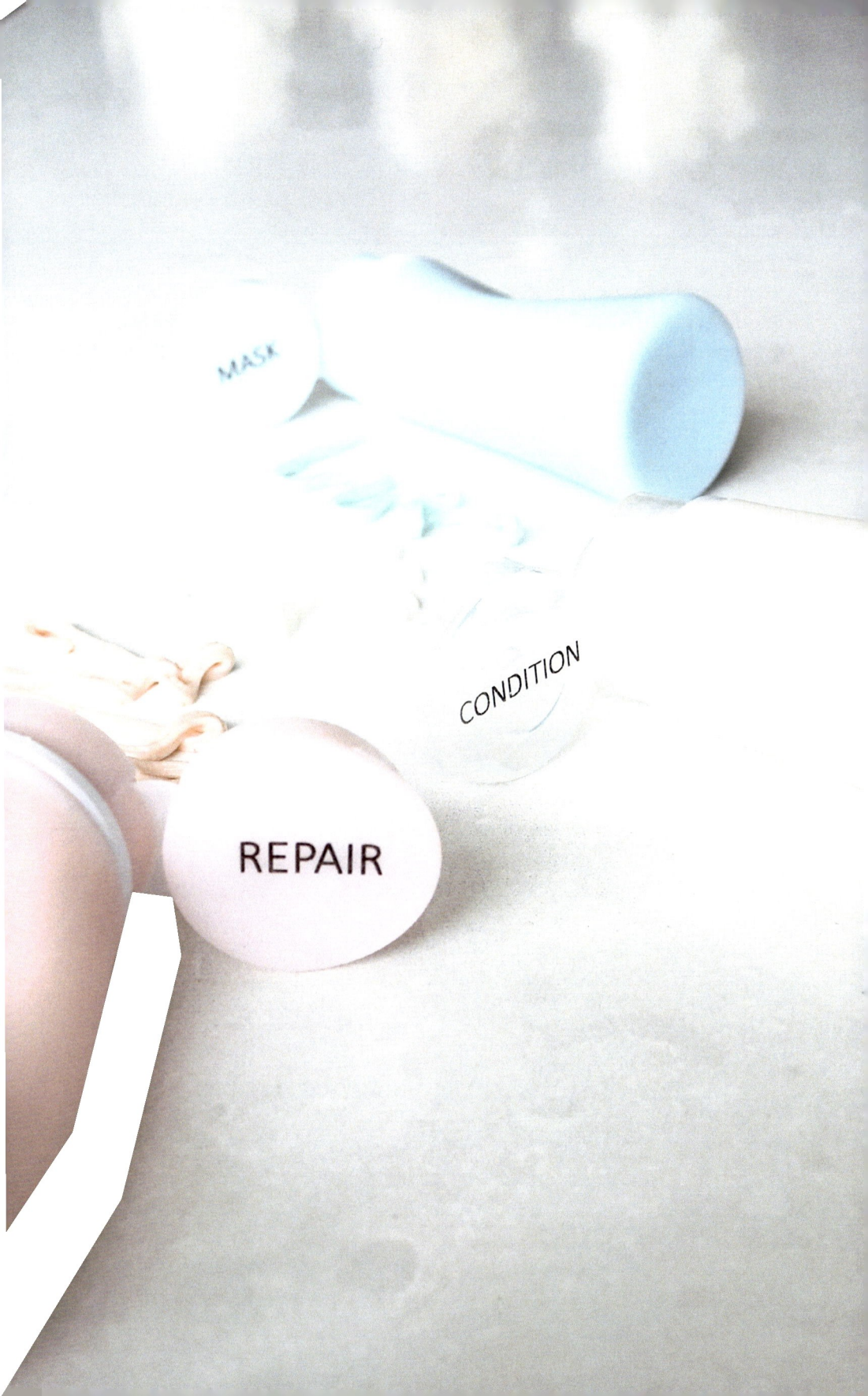

CONDITION

REPAIR

Honey Humectant Hair Conditioner

Honey extract has both emollient and humectant properties, making it a great hair moisturizer. Emollients smooth the hair follicles, adding shine to dull hair. Humectants bond with water molecules, adding moisture to dry strands. By moisturizing and locking in shine, honey can help restore the natural luster of your hair. Clary sage together with lavender essential oil can balance oil production and prevent itchy scalp.

Raw Ingredients:

15 g murumuru butter
10 ml argan oil
10 ml marula oil
10 ml macadamia nut oil
10 ml vegetable glycerin
7 g emulsifying wax
1 tsp honey superfood powder
110 ml distilled water
5 ml natural preservative
15 drops lavender essential oil
10 drops clary sage essential oil
2 drops vitamin E (MT-50)

Kitchen Tools:

You will need a double boiler, 2 metal pots, scale, 2 beakers, measuring spoons, spatula, whisk, and a jar or silicone bottle.

Recipe Prep Time

Prep Time: 15 minutes
Set Time: 30 minutes
Qty: 120 ml

Method:

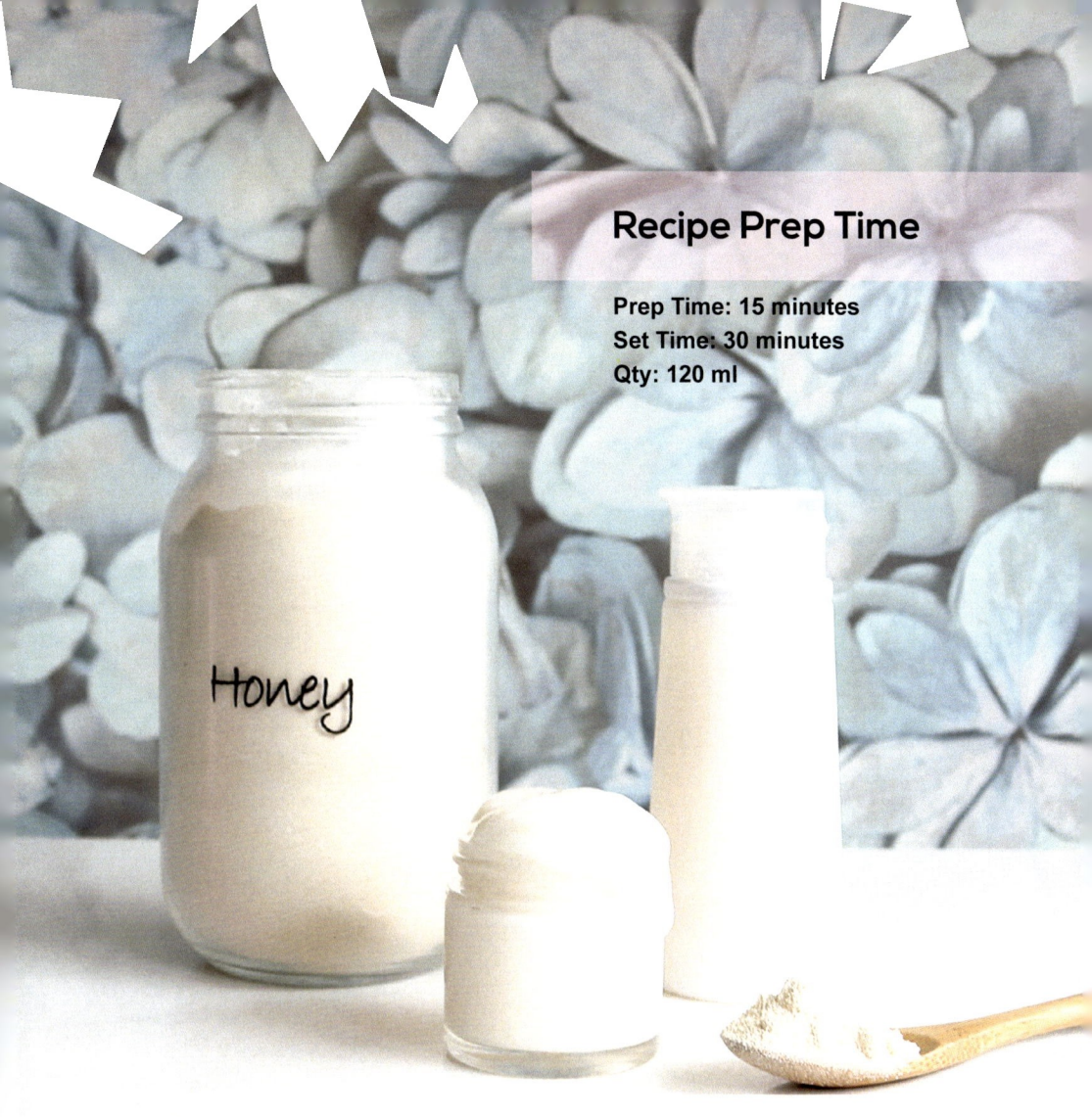

1. In a double boiler, gradually melt the butter. Add in the emulsifying wax (Pot 1).
2. Once melted, add in the carrier oils and vegetable glycerin (Pot 1).
3. In a separate pot (Pot 2), heat up the distilled water and add the honey superfood extract. Whisk.
4. Remove Pot 1 from heat and pour into a clean dry beaker or Pyrex (Beaker 1).
5. Remove Pot 2 from heat and pour in a SEPARATE clean dry beaker (Beaker 2).
6. Slowly pour Beaker 2 into Beaker 1, while whisking. This must be done slowly. Take about 2 minutes to complete this step.
7. Leave the mixture out on the counter to cool for about 3 minutes.
8. Add in the natural preservative, vitamin E and essential oils. Whisk well.
9. Continue whisking for about 5 minutes. It will become thicker as you whisk.
10. Pour mixture into your jar or a silicone bottle.
11. Pop in the fridge for about 30 minutes to set and thicken.

Raspberry Repair Protein Treatment

Frizzy or broken hair may need an extra dose of protein! This superfood repair cream is designed to reinforce the exterior structure of your hair, improving texture and strength. Infused with red raspberry extract, banana extract and broccoli seed oil, this bond-strengthening cream treats the outermost layer of the hair cuticle with natural proteins and essential amino acids. Bergamot helps reduce inflammation, promoting healthy hair growth and a healthy scalp.

Raw Ingredients:

5 g murumuru butter
5 g babassu butter
35 g carrot butter
1/2 tsp raspberry superfood powder
1/2 tsp banana superfood powder
20 ml olive oil
15 ml broccoli seed oil
1 tbsp extra virgin coconut oil
20 drops bergamot essential oil
1 drop vitamin e (MT-50)

Kitchen Tools:

You will need a double boiler, metal pot, scale, beaker, measuring spoons, spatula, whisk, an electric mixer and a jar or silicone bottle.

Recipe Prep Time

Prep Time: 15 minutes
Set Time: 30 minutes
Qty: 120 ml

Tip: This soft-serve cream can also be transferred to a squeezy silicone bottle using a piping bag. Perfect for travel.

Method:

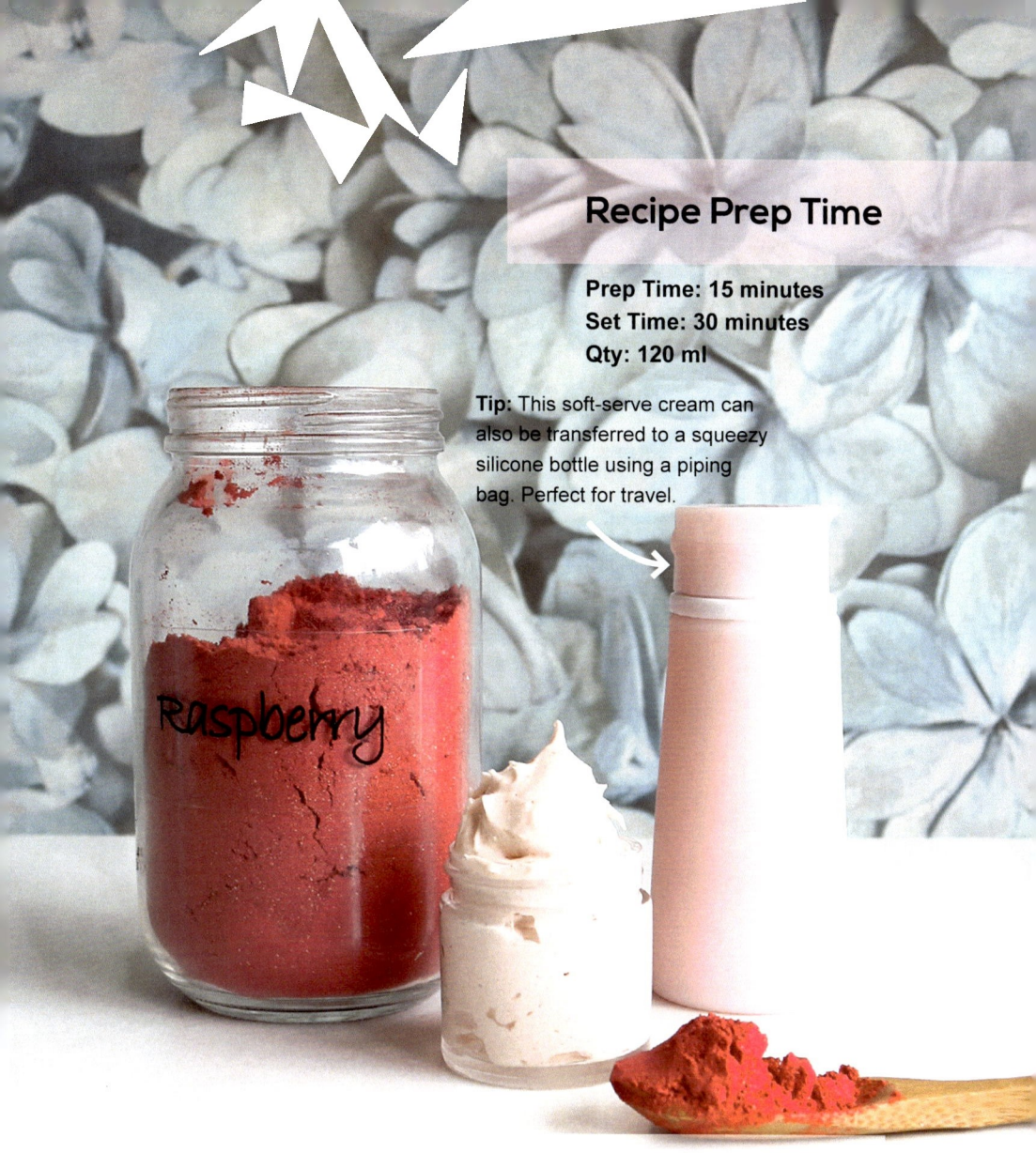

1. In a double boiler, gradually melt the 3 butters and extra virgin coconut oil.
2. Add in the carrier oils (olive, broccoli).
3. Once the butter and extra virgin coconut oil are melted, add in the superfood powders. Mix well.
4. Remove from heat and pour into a beaker or Pyrex.
5. Leave the mixture out on the counter to cool for about 3 minutes. Add in vitamin e and essential oils. Mix well.
6. Pop in the fridge for about 30 minutes or until semi-solid.
7. Fluff it up with an electric hand mixer.
8. Then transfer the mixture into a jar or silicone bottle.

Sky Blue Clay Hair Mask

This overnight hair mask treatment gently penetrates your hair cuticles while you sleep, so you can wake up with smoother, softer, and ridiculously shinier hair. Blue clay works its magic to repair and strengthen the hair follicle while antioxidant-rich murumuru hair butter delivers natural shine and gloss. Whipped and light weight.

Raw Ingredients:

5 g murumuru butter
5 g tucuma butter
35 g mango butter
20 ml argan oil
15 ml marula oil
1 tbsp extra virgin coconut oil
1 tsp blue clay
20 drops peppermint essential oil
1 drop vitamin E (MT-50)

Kitchen Tools:

You will need a double boiler, metal pot, scale, beaker (or Pyrex), measuring spoons, spatula, whisk, an electric mixer and a jar (silicone bottle is optional).

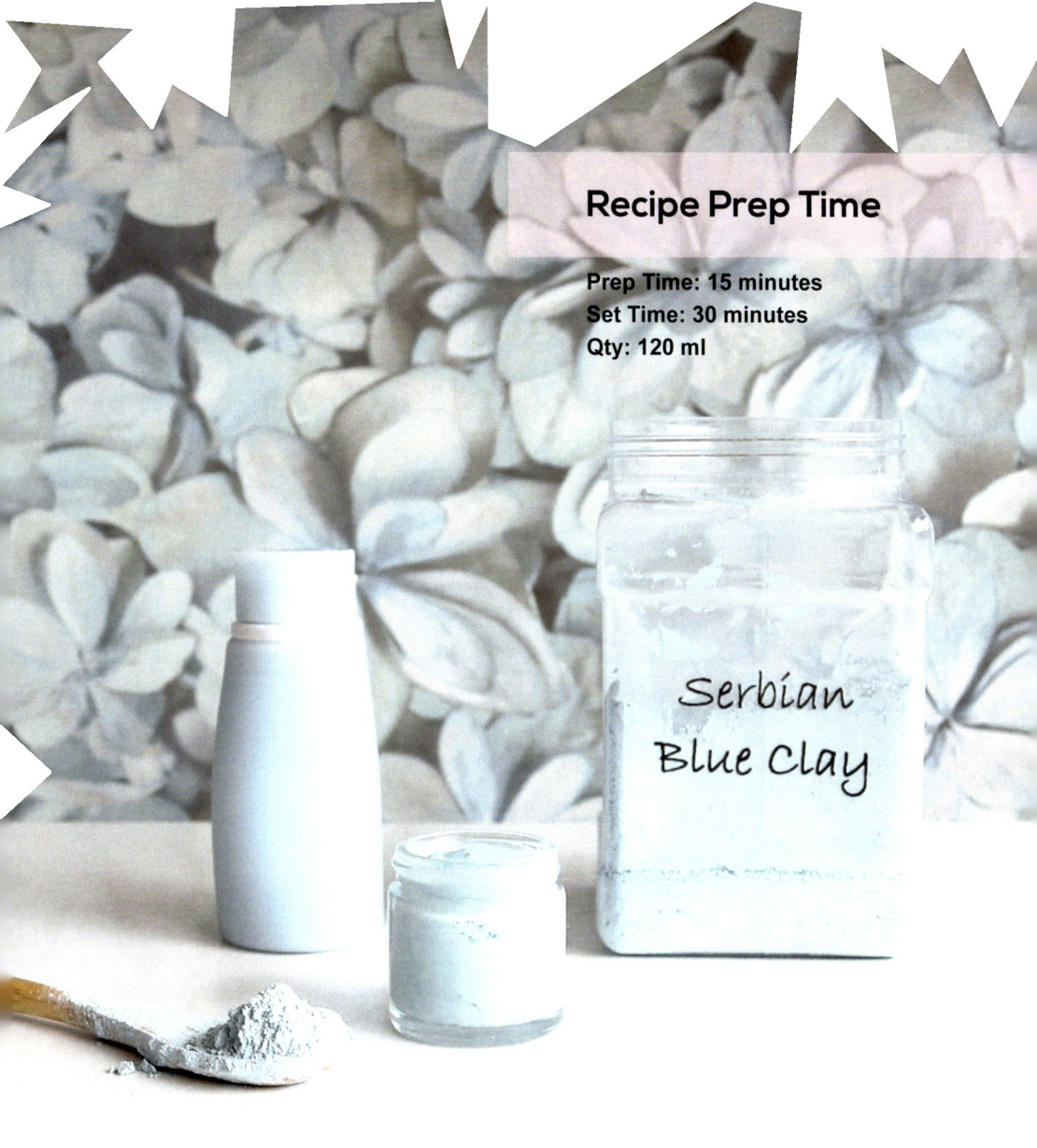

Recipe Prep Time

Prep Time: 15 minutes
Set Time: 30 minutes
Qty: 120 ml

Method:

1. In a double boiler, gradually melt the butters and extra virgin coconut oil.
2. Once melted, add in the carrier oils (argan, marula).
3. Add in the blue clay. Mix well.
4. Remove from heat and pour in a clean dry beaker or Pyrex.
5. Leave the mixture out on the counter to cool for about 3 minutes. Add in vitamin E and the essential oil. Whisk.
6. Pop in the fridge for about 30 minutes or until semi-solid.
7. Fluff it up with an electric hand mixer.
8. Then transfer the mixture into the jar.

Green Clay 2-in-1 Scalp + Shower Cleansing Bar (Oily Skin)

Give your skin and scalp a deep cleanse. Green clay purifies and detoxifies the scalp, removing dead skin cells and product build up, while aloe soothes and reduces inflammation. Rosemary oil's antimicrobial benefits help balance and tone the skin and scalp.

Raw Ingredients:

145 g aloe melt & pour soap base
1/2 tsp green clay
1/4 tsp rosemary superfood powder
12 drops grapefruit essential oil
8 drops rosemary essential oil

Kitchen Tools:

You will need a double boiler, Pyrex or small metal pot, scale, beaker, whisk, measuring spoon and a silicone mold.

Recipe Prep Time

Prep Time: 15 minutes
Set Time: 25 minutes
Qty: 145 g bar

To use: Gently massage the clay side of the bar onto your scalp in circular motions. Use weekly. Shampoo and condition afterwards. Use the soap side of the bar on your body in the shower.

Method:

1. In a double boiler, gradually melt the soap base.
2. Once melted transfer into the beaker.
3. Mix in the superfood extract, clay and essential oils.
4. Quickly pour the liquid evenly into the mold.
5. Carefully transfer the molds to the fridge for about 25 minutes to set faster.
6. Once the bars have solidified remove from mold.

To create a layered bar: At step 2, transfer half of the soap base into the beaker and add the essential oils. Mix well and then pour into your mold. Add your superfood powders and clay to the remaining soap base in your double boiler and mix well. Transfer into a beaker. Pour it over your first layer in the mold. Allow 2-5 minutes for the first layer to harden before pouring the second layer. Proceed to step 5.

Yellow Clay 2-in-1 Scalp + Shower Cleansing Bar (Normal Skin)

The all-natural scalp and body cleanser utilizes yellow clay to clean hair follicles so you can continue to grow thicker, healthy hair. Essential oils of chamomile and ylang ylang are suitable for normal to dry scalp and promote shinier hair. Honey offers moisturizing and antibacterial properties.

Raw Ingredients:

145 g honey melt & pour soap base
1/2 tsp yellow clay
1/4 tsp organic coconut milk superfood powder
15 drops chamomile essential oil
5 drops ylang ylang essential oil

Kitchen Tools:

You will need a double boiler, Pyrex or small metal pot, scale, beaker, whisk, measuring spoon and a silicone mold.

Recipe Prep Time

Prep Time: 15 minutes
Set Time: 25 minutes
Qty: 145 g bar

Method:

1. In a double boiler, gradually melt the soap base.
2. Once melted transfer into the beaker.
3. Mix in the superfood extract, clay and essential oils.
4. Quickly pour the liquid evenly into the mold.
5. Carefully transfer the molds to the fridge for about 25 minutes to set faster.
6. Once the bars have solidified remove from mold.

To create a layered bar: At step 2, transfer half of the soap base into the beaker and add the essential oils. Mix well and then pour into your mold. Add your superfood powders and clay to the remaining soap base in your double boiler and mix well. Pour it over your first layer in the mold. Allow 2-5 minutes for the first layer to harden before pouring the second layer. Proceed to step 5.

Pink Clay 2-in-1 Scalp + Shower Cleansing Bar (Dry Skin)

The perfect exfoliator and hydrator for your scalp and body. This recipe targets dry and sensitive skin types. Pink clay reduces irritation and inflammation on the skin and gently exfoliates flaky skin. Shea is ultra hydrating on the skin. Geranium essential oil balances the pH of your skin while sandalwood reduces irritation.

Raw Ingredients:

145 g shea melt & pour soap base
1/2 tsp pink clay
1/4 tsp beet root superfood powder
12 drops sandalwood essential oil
8 drops geranium essential oil

Kitchen Tools:

You will need a double boiler, Pyrex or small metal pot, scale, beaker, whisk, measuring spoon and a silicone mold.

Recipe Prep Time

Prep Time: 15 minutes
Set Time: 25 minutes
Qty: 145 g bar

Method:

1. In a double boiler, gradually melt the soap base.
2. Once melted transfer into the beaker.
3. Mix in the superfood extract, clay and essential oils.
4. Quickly pour the liquid evenly into the mold.
5. Carefully transfer the molds to the fridge for about 25 minutes to set faster.
6. Once the bars have solidified remove from mold.

To create a layered bar: At step 2, transfer half of the soap base into the beaker and add the essential oils. Mix well and then pour into your mold. Add your superfood powders and clay to the remaining soap base in your double boiler and mix well. Pour it over your first layer in the mold. Allow 2-5 minutes for the first layer to harden before pouring the second layer. Proceed to step 5.

Papaya-Bergamot Scalp + Body Clay Scrub

Goodbye itchy, flaky, dry scalp! Papaya enzymes and Dead Sea Salt work to prevent oil build-up on the scalp, which often causes problems like dandruff and dermatitis.

Raw Ingredients:

600 g dead sea salt (ultra fine, not too coarse)
60 ml fractionated coconut oil
35 g extra virgin coconut oil
1/2 tsp kaolin white clay
1/2 tsp papaya superfood powder
10 drops broccoli seed oil
10 drops marula oil
30 drops bergamot essential oil

Kitchen Tools:

You will need a large bowl, spatula, scale, measuring spoons and a jar.

Recipe Prep Time

Prep Time: 10 minutes
Set Time: 10 minutes
Qty: 500 g jar

Shower Ritual: Massage a handful onto damp skin and damp scalp in the shower or bath using circular motions. Allow the product and salts to work their magic about 1 minute before rinsing out. Shampoo and condition as per usual.

Method:

1. Pour mineral salt into a clean bowl.
2. Add in extra virgin coconut oil.
3. "Wet" the salt with the carrier oils (broccoli, marula, fractionated coconut oil).
4. Sprinkle in the superfood extract and clay.
5. Add in the essential oil.
6. Using a spatula, mix all ingredients together.
7. Hand pack in a jar.

Sweet Potato-Eucalyptus Scalp + Body Clay Scrub

Try this recipe for a much needed scalp and skin detox. Sweet Potato extract is a rich source of magnesium and beta-carotene that aids in cell growth and can prevent hair thinning and even reduce dullness in hair. Invigorating essential oils of eucalyptus and wintergreen are stimulating and help to improve blood circulation.

Raw Ingredients:

600 g dead sea salt (ultra fine, not too coarse)
60 ml fractionated coconut oil
35 g extra virgin coconut oil
1/2 tsp kaolin white clay
1/2 tsp sweet potato superfood powder
10 drops broccoli seed oil
10 drops marula oil
20 drops eucalyptus essential oil
10 drops wintergreen essential oil

Kitchen Tools:

You will need a large bowl, spatula, scale, measuring spoons and a jar.

Recipe Prep Time

Prep Time: 10 minutes
Set Time: 10 minutes
Qty: 500 g jar

Method:

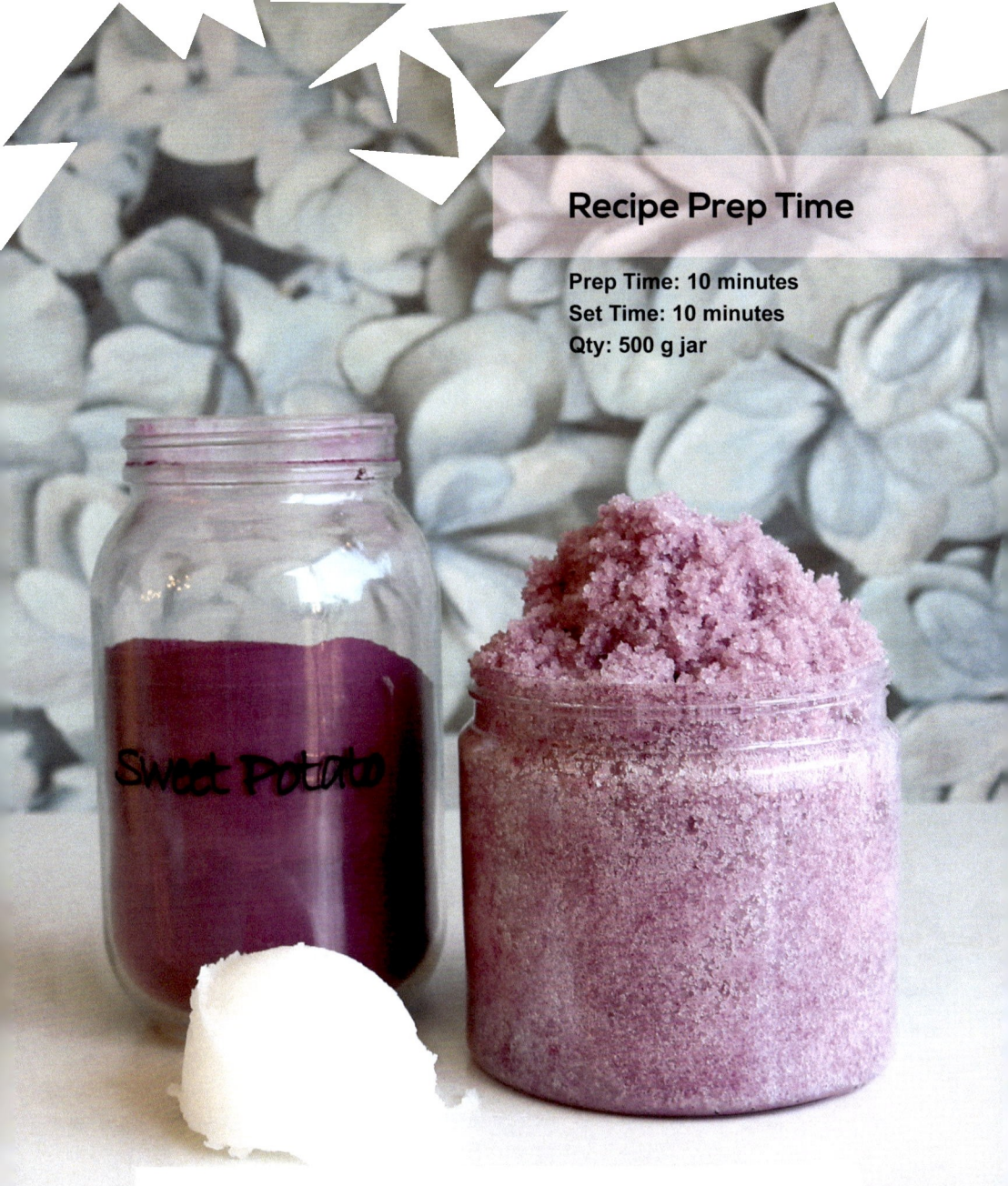

1. Pour mineral salt into a clean bowl.
2. Add in extra virgin coconut oil.
3. "Wet" the salt with the carrier oils.
4. Sprinkle in the sweet potato superfood powder and clay.
5. Add in the essential oils.
6. Using a spatula, mix all ingredients together.
7. Hand pack in a jar.

Broccoli Scalp Serum Treatment

Boost your hair health with Broccoli oil! It adds moisturizing fatty acids and vitamins that are essential to healthy hair growth. Essential oils of cedarwood balance the oil-producing glands in the scalp and lemongrass can help strengthen the hair follicles.

Raw Ingredients:

15 ml grape seed oil
10 ml broccoli seed oil
5 ml hemp seed oil
10 drops cedarwood essential oil
5 drops lemongrass essential oil
1 drop vitamin E (MT-50)

Kitchen Tools:

You will need a funnel and a bottle.

Recipe Prep Time

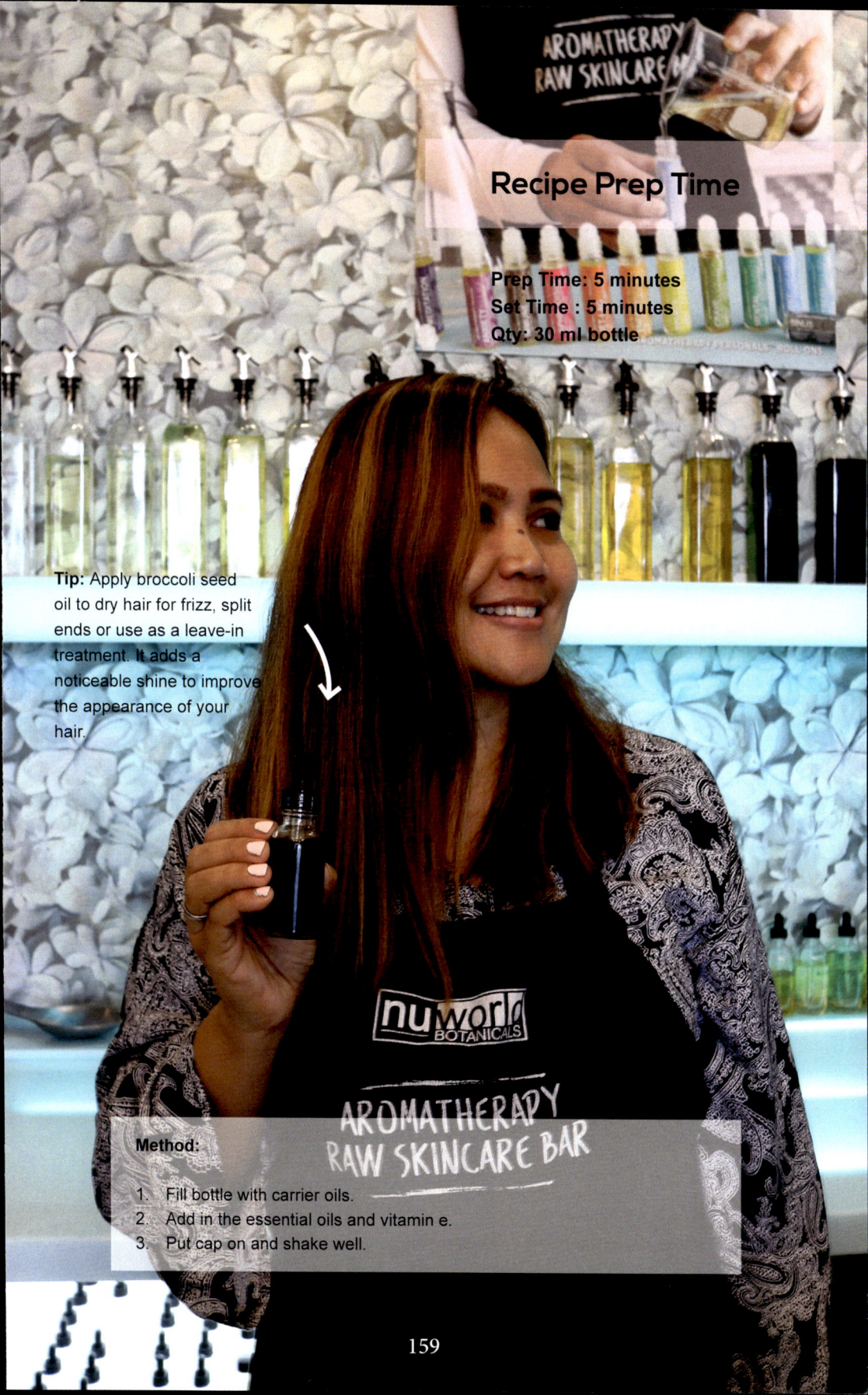

Prep Time: 5 minutes
Set Time : 5 minutes
Qty: 30 ml bottle

Tip: Apply broccoli seed oil to dry hair for frizz, split ends or use as a leave-in treatment. It adds a noticeable shine to improve the appearance of your hair.

Method:

1. Fill bottle with carrier oils.
2. Add in the essential oils and vitamin e.
3. Put cap on and shake well.

DIY Superfood Bronzer Recipes

It's all about the sun-kissed glow.

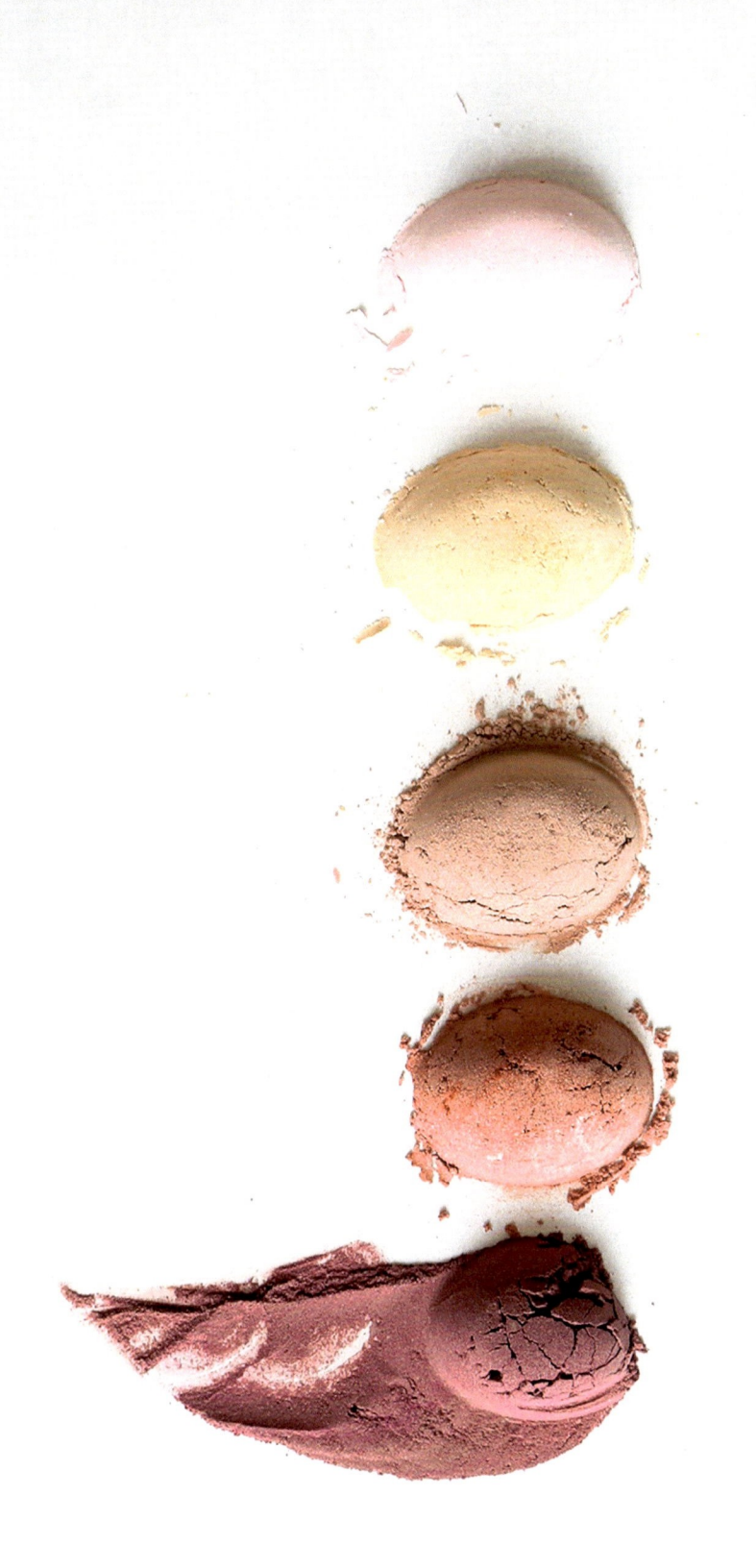

Pink Watermelon Highlighting Mineral Powder

This pink pearlescent blend adds highlights right where you need them for a subtle shimmer and glow! This light-reflective powder not only gives your skin shimmering pink highlights, it's ultra-rich in vitamin C and minerals.

Raw Ingredients:

2 1/2 tsp arrowroot powder
1 1/8 tsp organic coconut superfood powder
1 1/8 tsp pink clay
2 tsp pink mineral mica powder
1 tsp pearl mineral mica powder
1/4 tsp watermelon superfood powder
1/4 tsp hibiscus superfood powder
1/4 tsp raspberry superfood powder
1/4 tsp guava superfood powder

Kitchen Tools:

You will need a bowl, spoon, whisk, measuring spoon and a powder jar.

Recipe Prep Time

Prep Time: 5 minutes
Set Time: 5 minutes
Qty: 30 g jar

To Use: Tap a powder brush into the powder then sweep it along your cheekbones and around the perimeter of your face, like your temples and forehead—basically all the places where the sun typically hits.

Method:

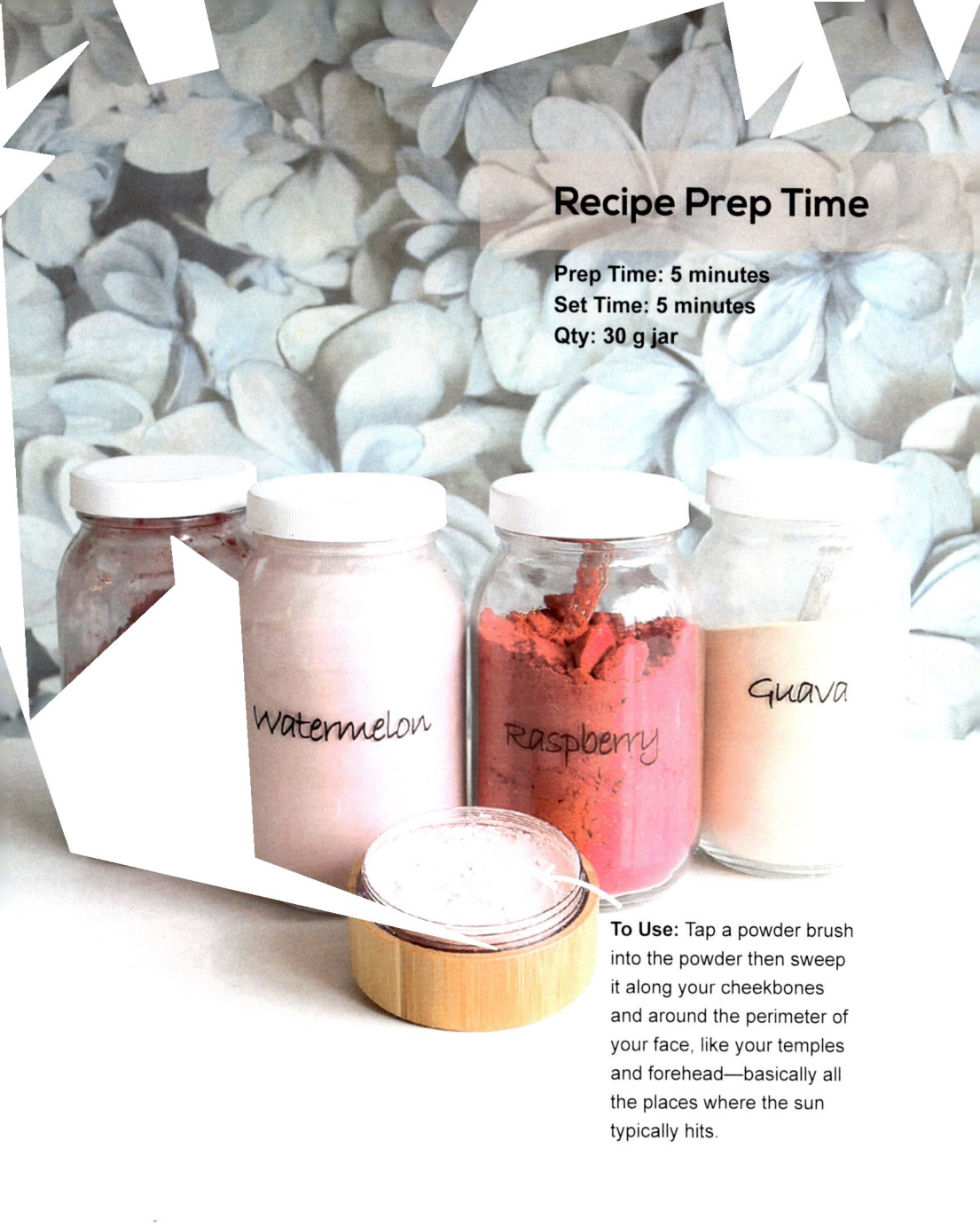

1. In a mixing bowl, add in arrowroot powder and organic coconut powder. Whisk.
2. Add in the superfood extracts, mineral mica powders and clay. Whisk well.
3. Using a spoon, transfer the dry powder mixture to your jar.

Golden Pumpkin Bronzing Powder

Get that vacation glow and bring out your inner sun goddess! This luminous recipe pairs tropical fruits with vitamin c rich sea buckthorn for 8 hours of glowing skin.

Raw Ingredients:

2 1/2 tsp arrowroot powder
1 1/8 tsp organic coconut superfood powder
1 1/8 tsp yellow clay
2 tsp gold mineral mica powder
1 tsp pearl mineral mica powder
1/4 tsp pumpkin superfood powder
1/4 tsp sea buckthorn superfood powder
1/4 tsp papaya superfood powder
1/4 tsp mango superfood powder

Kitchen Tools:

You will need a bowl, spoon, whisk, measuring spoon and a powder jar.

Recipe Prep Time

Prep Time: 5 minutes
Set Time: 5 minutes
Qty: 30 g jar

Method:

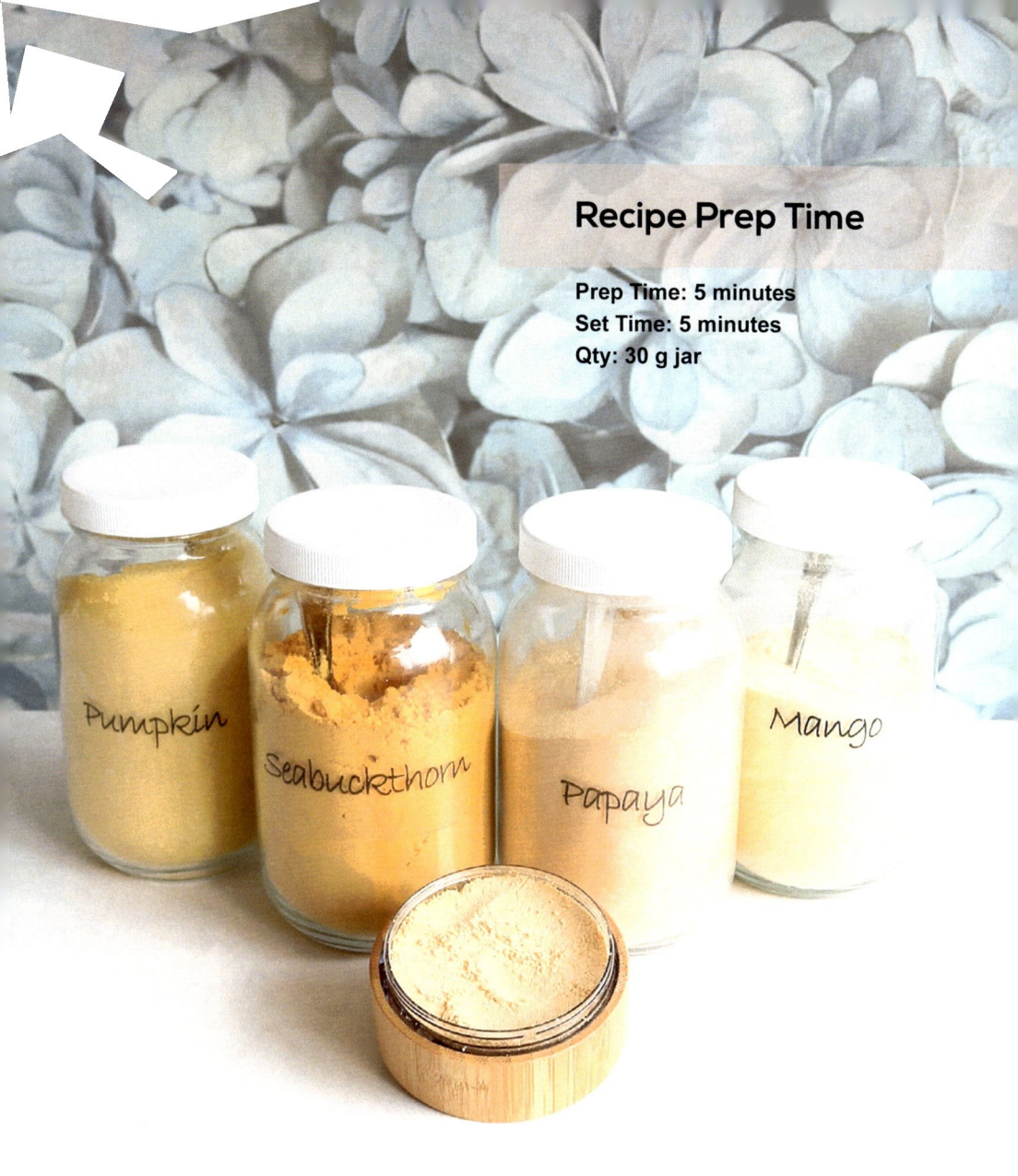

1. In a mixing bowl, add in arrowroot powder and organic coconut powder. Whisk.
2. Add in the superfood extracts, mineral mica powders and clay. Whisk.
3. Using a spoon, transfer the dry powder mixture to your jar.

Cranberry Copper Bronzing Powder (warm undertones)

These beautiful sun-kissed superfoods will add depth and warmth to your skin. The shimmer reflects light with a warm copper undertone and the skin-boosting superfoods deliver mega antioxidants. Coconut powder and rhassoul clay have sebum controlling minerals and can absorb surface oil throughout the day.

Raw Ingredients:

2 1/2 tsp arrowroot powder
1 1/8 tsp organic coconut superfood powder
1 1/8 tsp rhassoul clay
2 tsp copper mineral mica powder
1 tsp pearl mineral mica powder
1/4 tsp cranberry superfood powder
1/4 tsp strawberry superfood powder
1/4 tsp beet root superfood powder
1/4 tsp turmeric superfood powder

Kitchen Tools:

You will need a bowl, spoon, whisk, measuring spoon and a jar.

This strawberry powder ingredient makes our bronzer naturally smell like fresh strawberries!

Recipe Prep Time

Prep Time: 5 minutes
Set Time: 5 minutes
Qty: 30 g jar

Method:

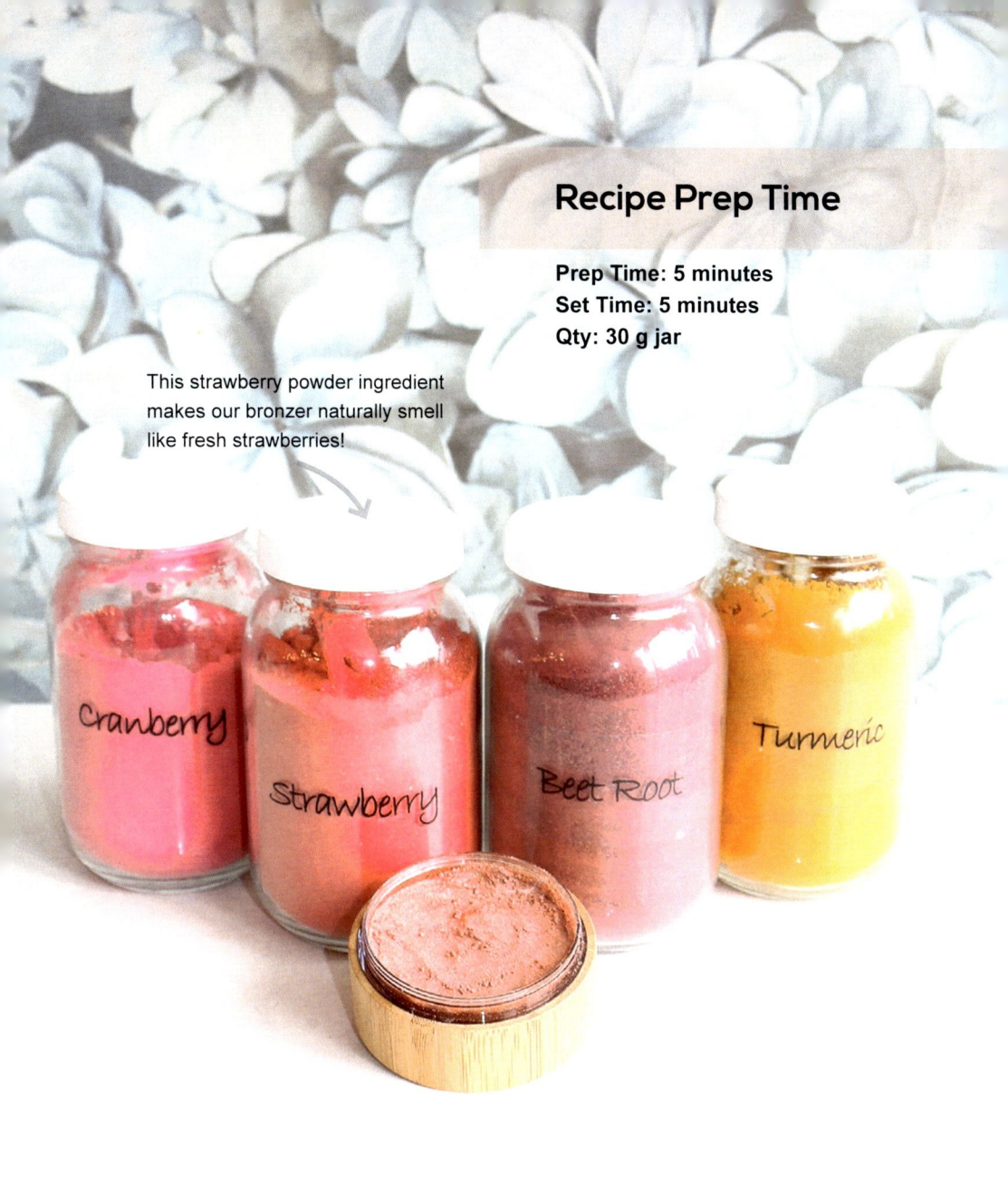

1. In a mixing, bowl add in arrowroot powder and organic coconut powder. Whisk.
2. Add in the superfood extracts, mineral mica powders and clay. Whisk.
3. Using a spoon, transfer the dry powder mixture to your jar.

Plum Potato Bronzing Powder (cool undertones)

Blue and purple superfoods like elderberry and sweet potato work well for cooler undertones plus they're packed with natural antioxidants for instant free radical protection. Arrowroot powder has anti-irritant and anti-inflammatory properties.

Raw Ingredients:

2 1/2 tsp arrowroot powder
1 1/8 tsp organic coconut superfood powder
1 1/8 tsp olive clay
2 tsp merlot mineral mica powder
1 tsp mahogany mineral mica powder
1/4 tsp butterfly pea superfood powder
1/4 tsp blue spirulina superfood powder
1/4 tsp elderberry superfood powder
1/4 tsp sweet potato superfood powder

Kitchen Tools:

You will need a bowl, spoon, whisk, measuring spoon and a powder jar.

Recipe Prep Time

Prep Time: 5 minutes
Set Time: 5 minutes
Qty: 30 g jar

Method:

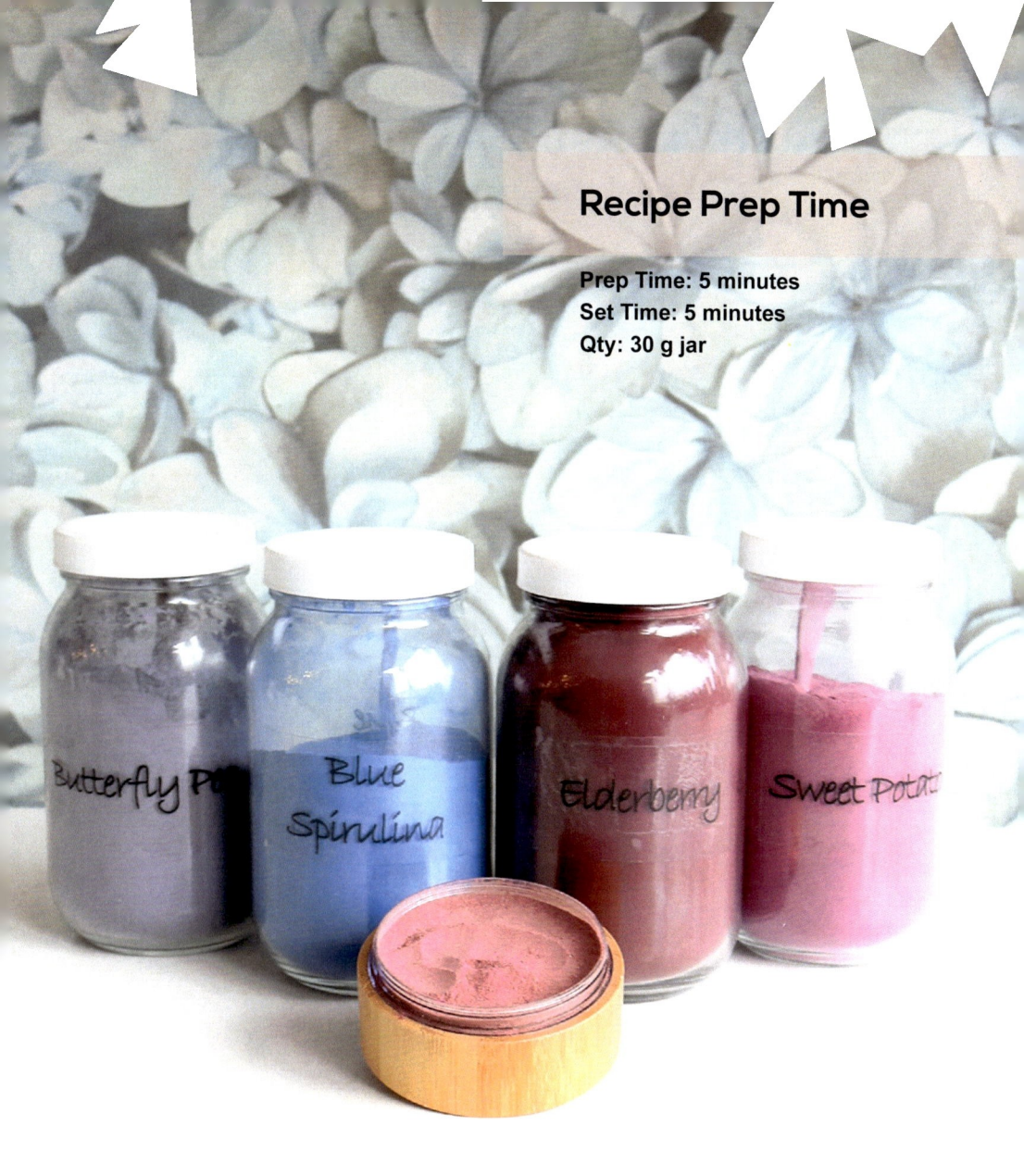

1. In a mixing bowl, add in arrowroot powder and organic coconut powder. Whisk.
2. Add in the superfood extracts, mineral mica powders and clay. Whisk.
3. Using a spoon, transfer the dry powder mixture to your jar.

Cocoa-Bamboo Bronzing Powder (neutral skin tones)

Not only is bamboo extract powder a gorgeous neutral shade, it's rich in silica content which gives your skin a radiant glow. It's also hydrating and packed with antimicrobial and anti-inflammatory properties.

Raw Ingredients:

2 1/2 tsp arrowroot powder
1 1/8 tsp organic coconut superfood powder
1 1/8 tsp rhassoul clay
2 tsp bronze mineral mica powder
1 tsp mahogany mineral mica powder
1/4 tsp bamboo leaf superfood powder
1/4 cocoa superfood powder
1/4 tsp golden berry superfood powder
1/4 tsp banana superfood powder

Kitchen Tools:

You will need a bowl, spoon, whisk, measuring spoon and a jar.

Recipe Prep Time

Prep Time: 5 minutes
Set Time: 5 minutes
Qty: 30 g jar

The best part about this recipe is that it smells just like chocolate!

Tip: If you like a contoured look, you can also run your powder brush along the edge of your jawline to define it. The key is to blend it out, and then blend some more.

Method:

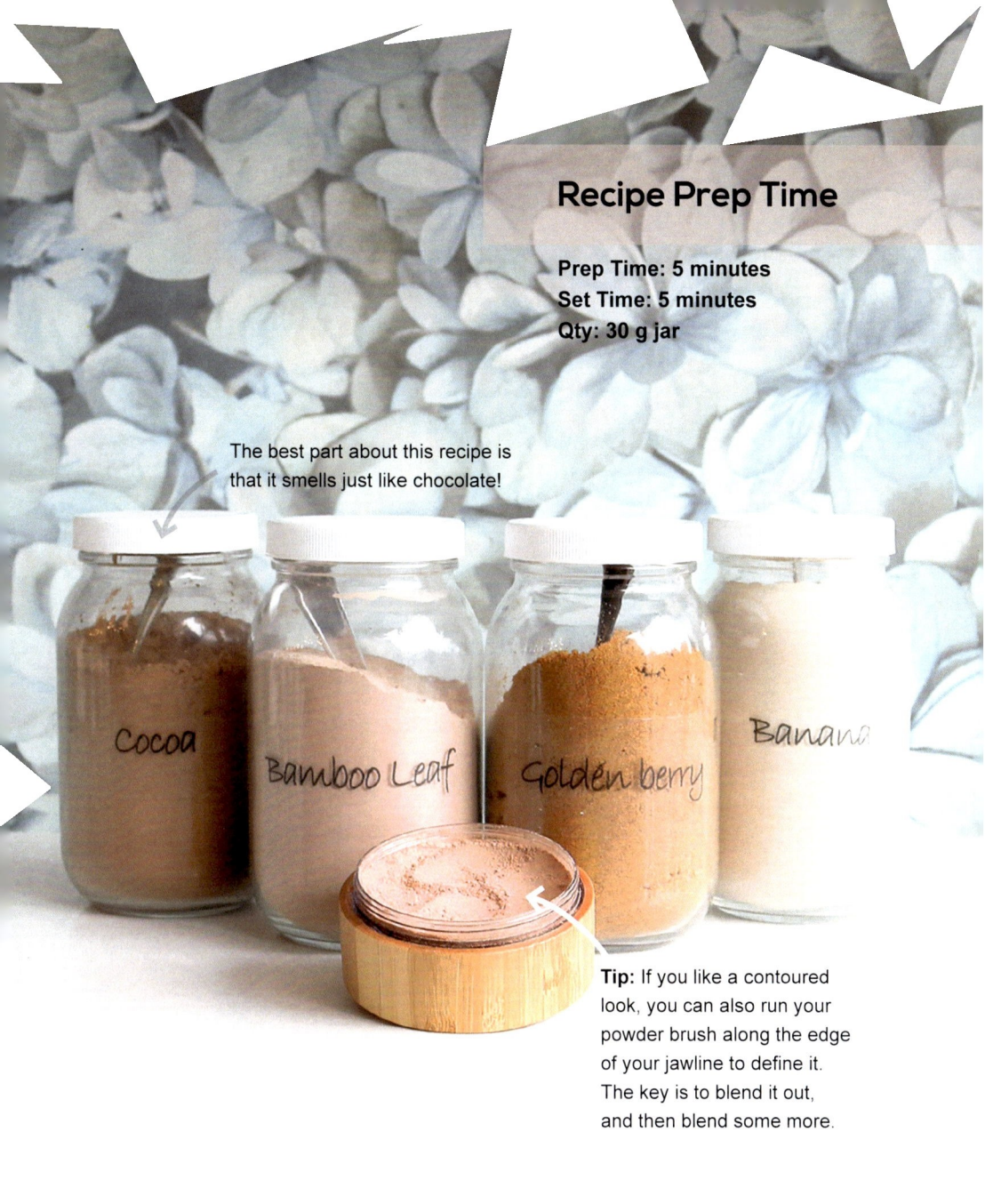

1. In a mixing bowl, add in arrowroot powder and organic coconut powder. Whisk.
2. Add in the superfood extracts, mineral mica powders and clay. Whisk.
3. Using a spoon, transfer the dry powder mixture to your jar.

Bronze-Nude Lip Gloss Luminizer + Highlighter

This hydrating warm toned formula is the ultimate 3-in-1 product that leaves lips feeling nourished. Perfect for use on lips, cheeks and as an eye gloss over the lids. For use on cheeks place one dot of gloss on the apple of your cheeks then blend away towards your ear.

Raw Ingredients:

10 ml vegetable glycerin
3.25 ml calendula carrier oil
1 tsp bronze mineral mica powder
1/4 tsp pearl mineral mica powder
1/8 tsp copper mineral mica powder
1/8 tsp mahogany mineral mica powder

Kitchen Tools:

You will need a bowl, whisk, measuring spoons, spoon, piping bag and a lip gloss tube.

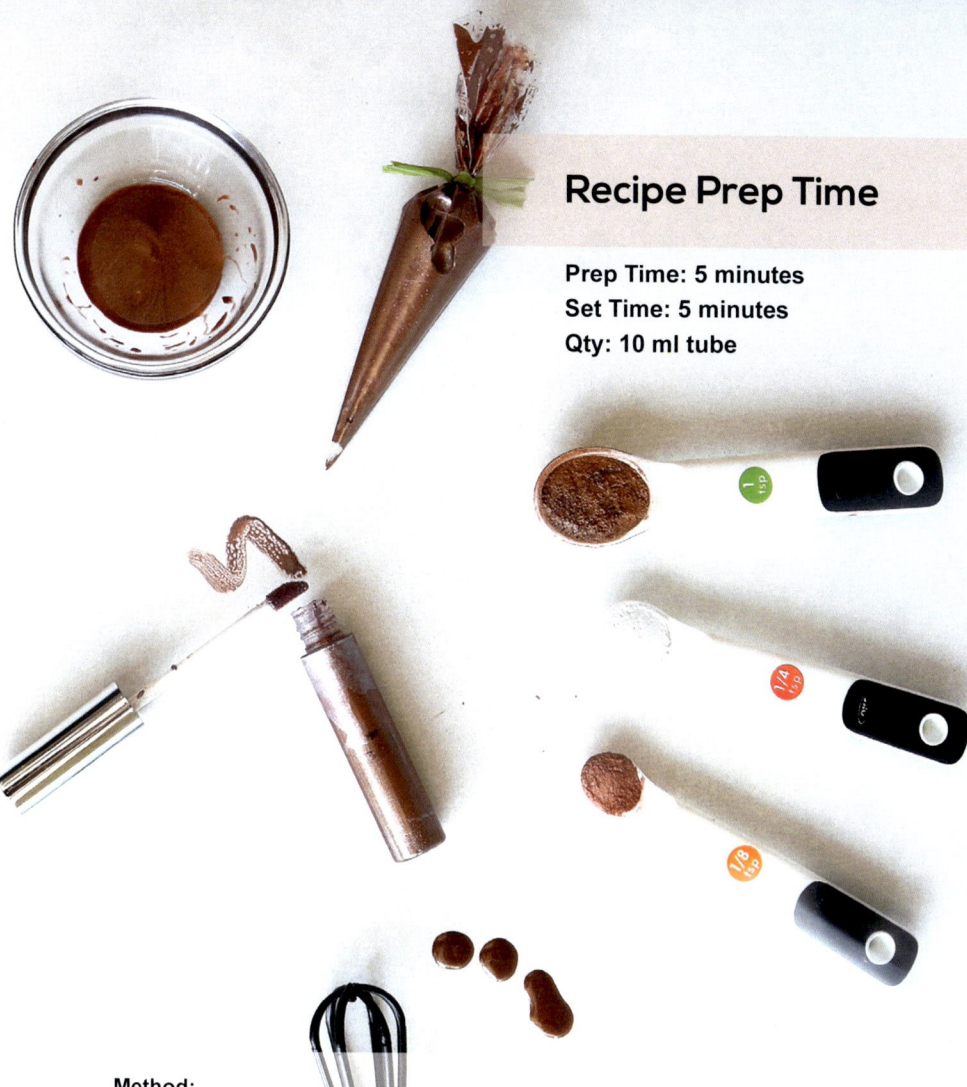

Recipe Prep Time

Prep Time: 5 minutes
Set Time: 5 minutes
Qty: 10 ml tube

Method:

1. In a small bowl, combine all of the dry mica powder ingredients. Using a whisk, mix well until combined.
2. Pour in the liquid ingredients (vegetable glycerine and oil). Continue to mix well with a whisk until it's combined well.
3. Using a spoon, scoop the lip gloss mixture from the bowl in towards the tip of the piping bag. DO NOT cut the tip of the bag until all of the mixture is in the bag.
4. Use scissors to cut a small opening at the end of the piping bag and insert the bag into the empty lip gloss tube.
5. Squeeze the mixture into the lip gloss tube.
6. Pop on the small plastic lip gloss plug.
7. Insert your lip gloss wand into the tube. Move the wand around and up and down a few times to remove any air bubbles.

Blush Pink Lip Gloss Luminizer + Highlighter

Give your lips a beautiful burst of pink colour and make your skin look healthy and glowy! Just a few dabs of this luminizer can brighten up your entire face—lips, brow bone and cheeks.

Raw Ingredients:

10 ml vegetable glycerin
3.25 ml carrier oil (ie. raspberry, calendula oil)
1 tsp hot pink mineral mica powder
3/8 tsp pearl mineral mica powder
1/8 tsp copper mineral mica powder

Kitchen Tools:

You will need a bowl, whisk, measuring spoons, spoon, piping bag and a lip gloss tube.

Recipe Prep Time

Prep Time: 5 minutes **Set Time:** 5 minutes
Qty: 10 ml tube

DIY Kit: Check out our pre-portioned DIY Lip Luminizer Kit. It includes everything you see here.

Method:

1. In a small bowl, combine all of the dry mica powder ingredients. Using a whisk, mix well until combined.
2. Pour in the liquid ingredients (vegetable glycerine and oil). Continue to mix well with a whisk until it's combined well.
3. Using a spoon, scoop the lip gloss mixture from the bowl in towards the tip of the piping bag. DO NOT cut the tip of the bag until all of the mixture is in the bag.
4. Use scissors to cut a small opening at the end of the piping bag and insert the bag into the empty lip gloss tube.
5. Squeeze the mixture into the lip gloss tube.
6. Pop on the small plastic lip gloss plug.
7. Insert your lip gloss wand into the tube. Move the wand around and up and down a few times to remove any air bubbles.

RAW CANDLE BAR

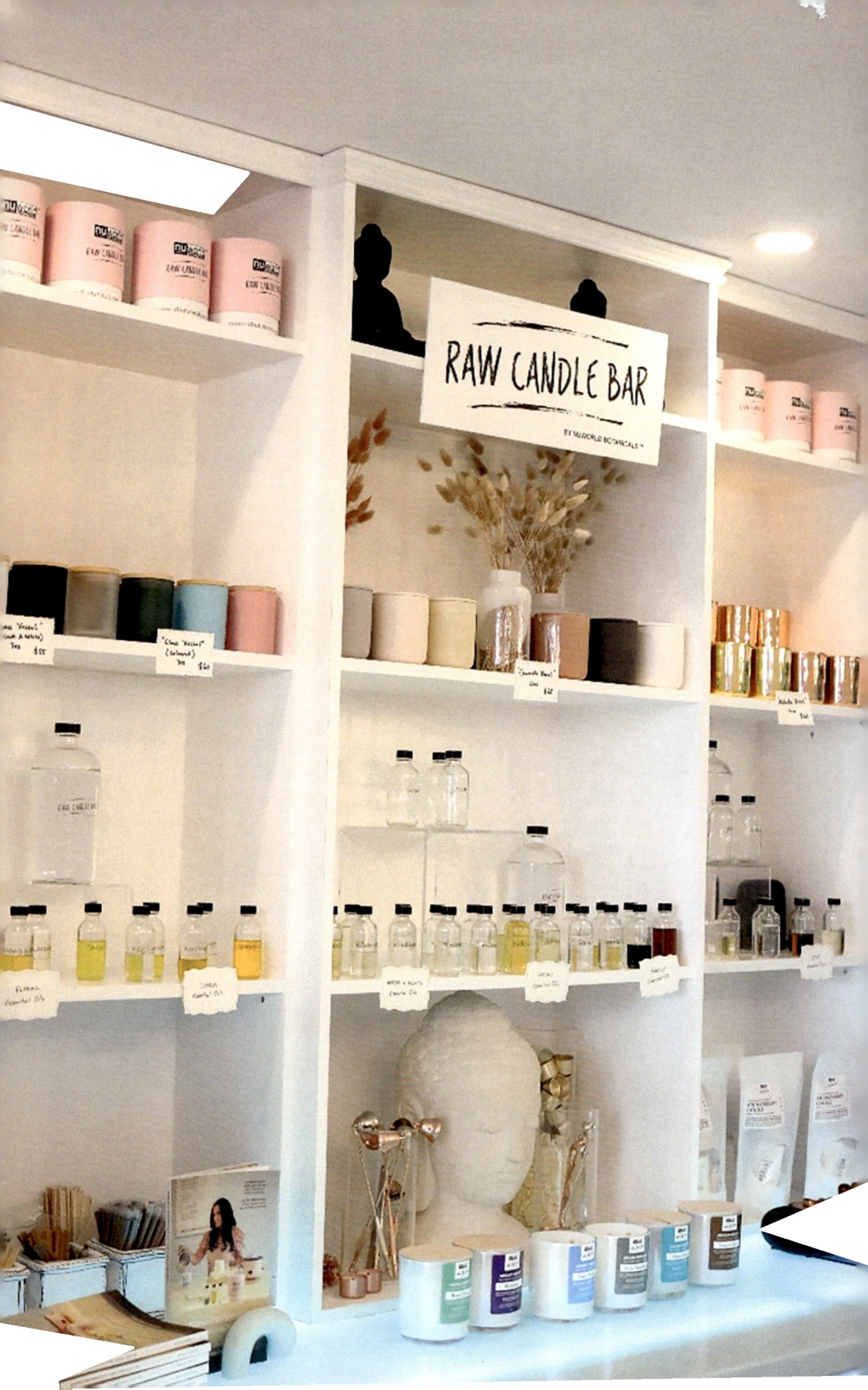

BY NUWORLD BOTANICALS

Reserved

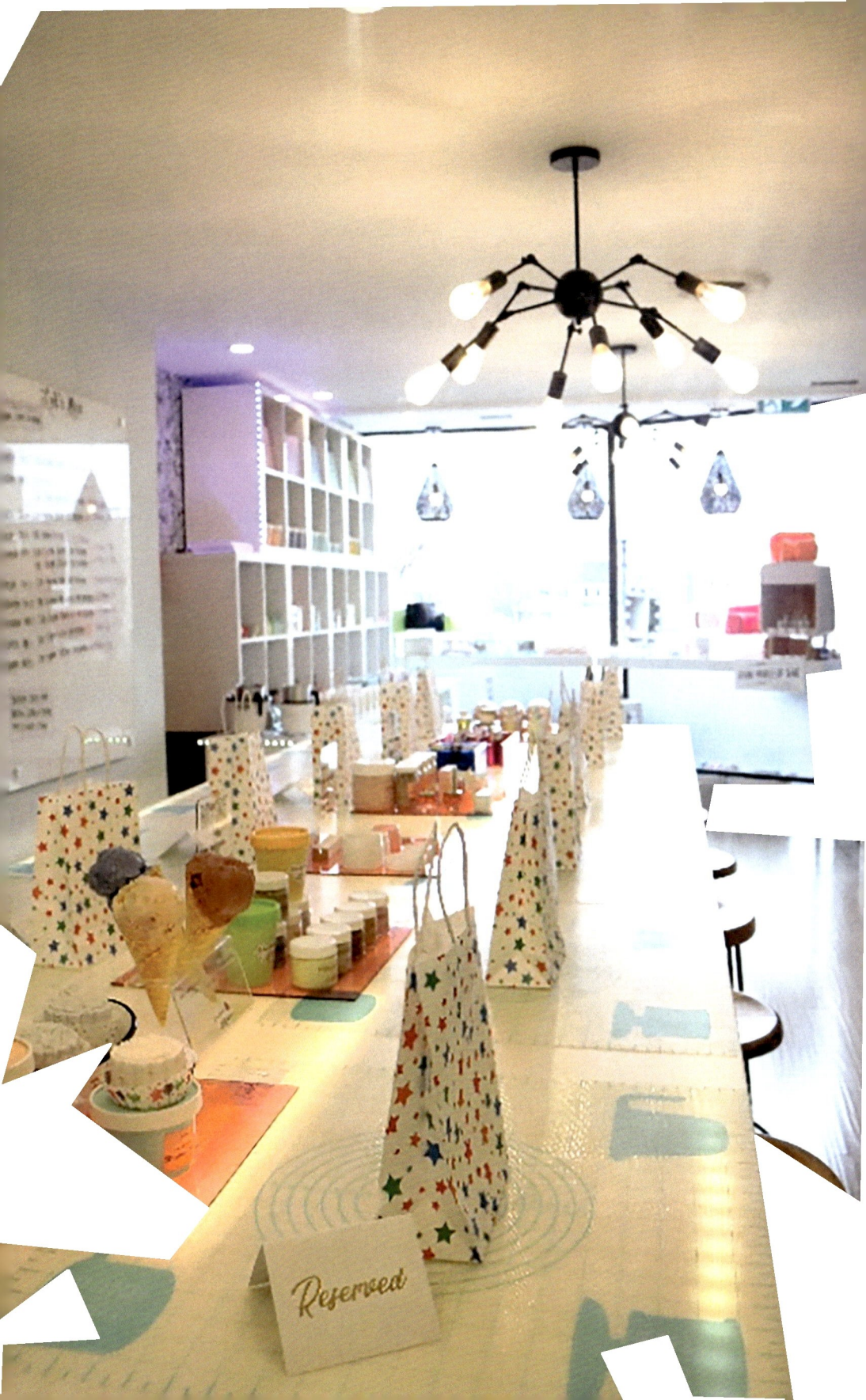

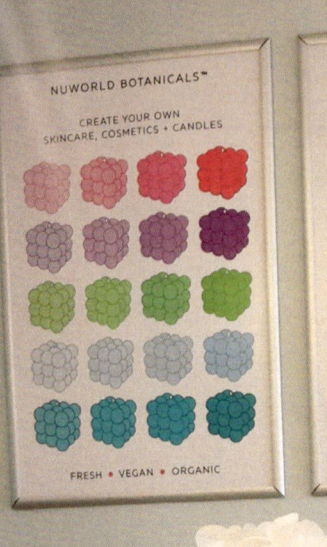

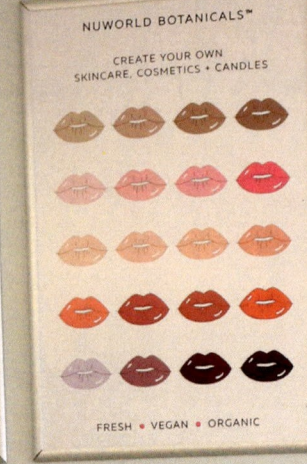

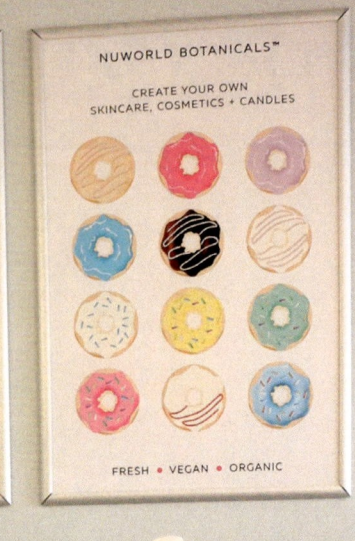

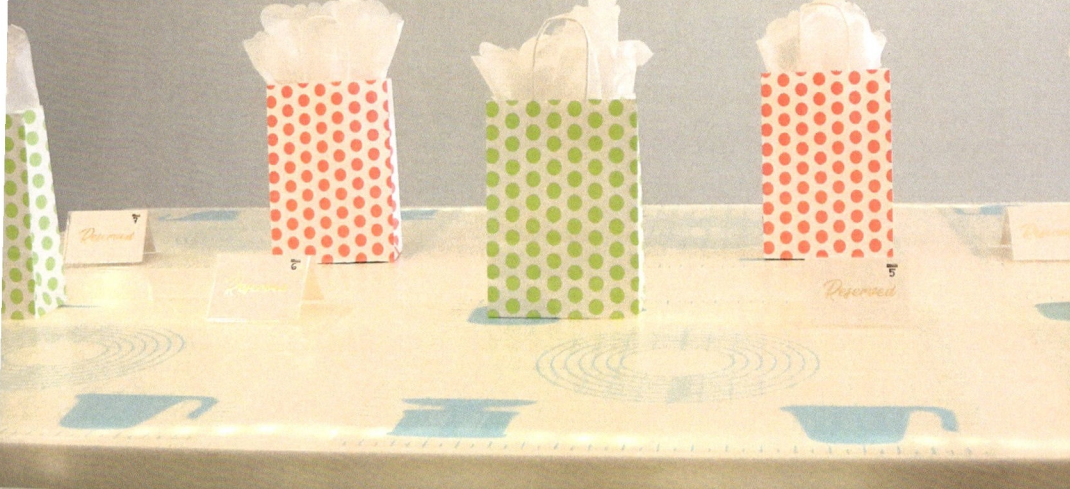

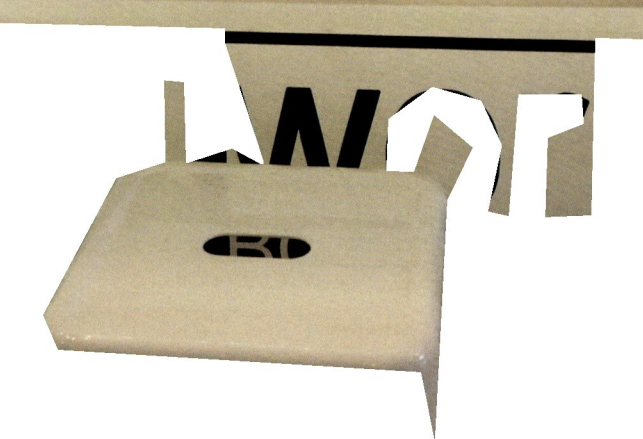

NUWORLD BOTANICALS
CREATE YOUR OWN
SKINCARE, COSMETICS + CANDLES

FRESH • VEGAN • ORGANIC

NUWORLD BOTANICALS
CREATE YOUR OWN
SKINCARE, COSMETICS + CANDLES

FRESH • VEGAN • ORGANIC

NUWORLD BOTANICALS
CREATE YOUR OWN
SKINCARE, COSMETICS + CANDLES

FRESH • VEGAN • ORGANIC

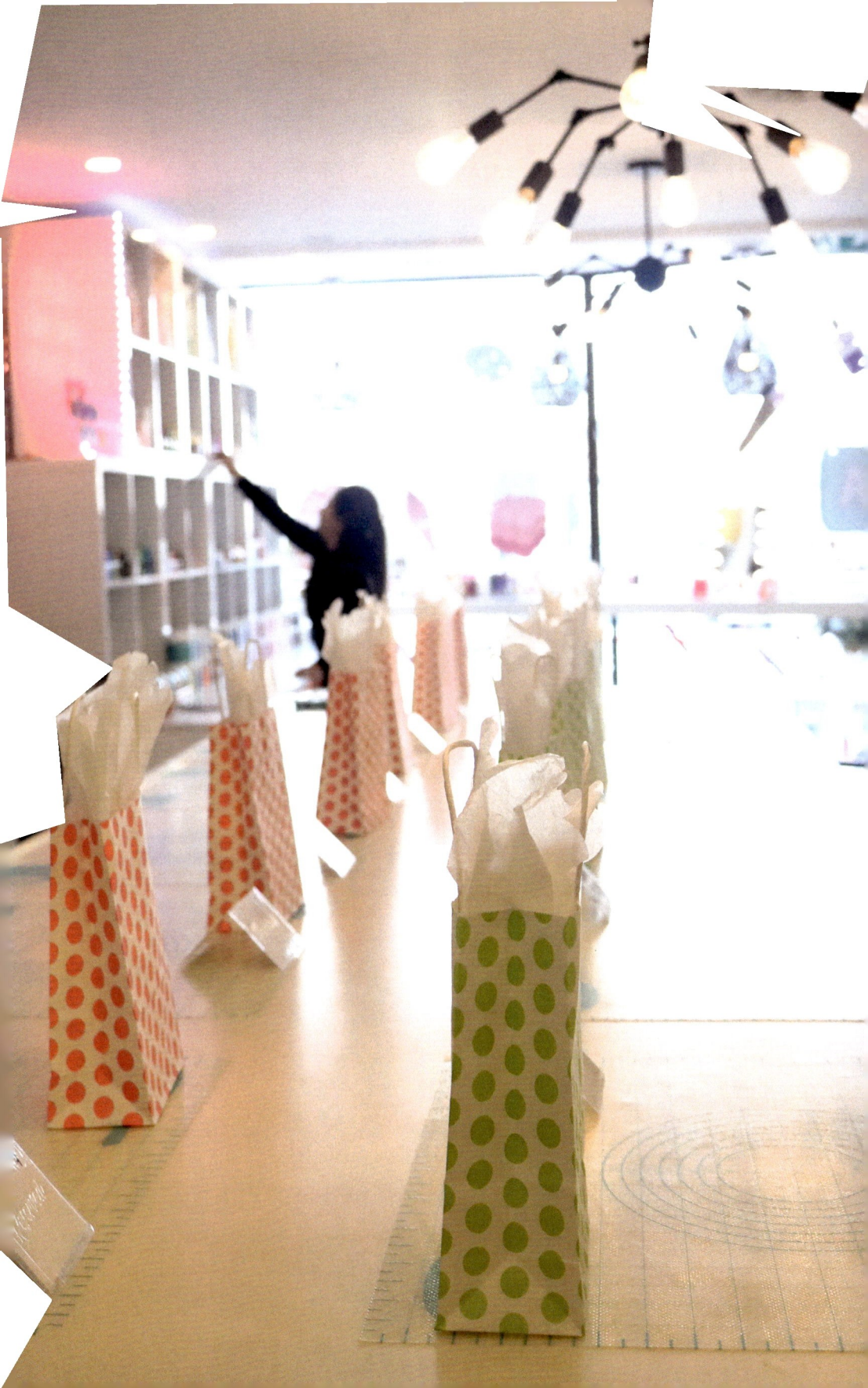

Fresh

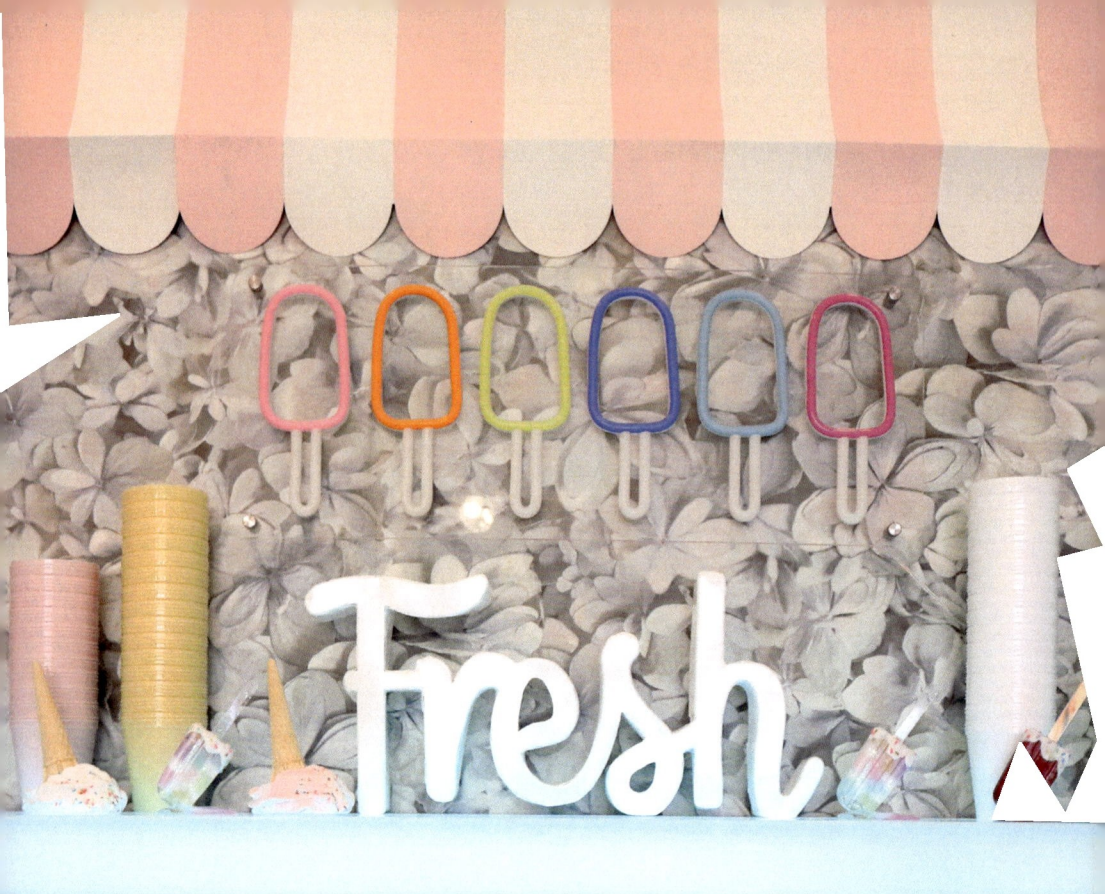

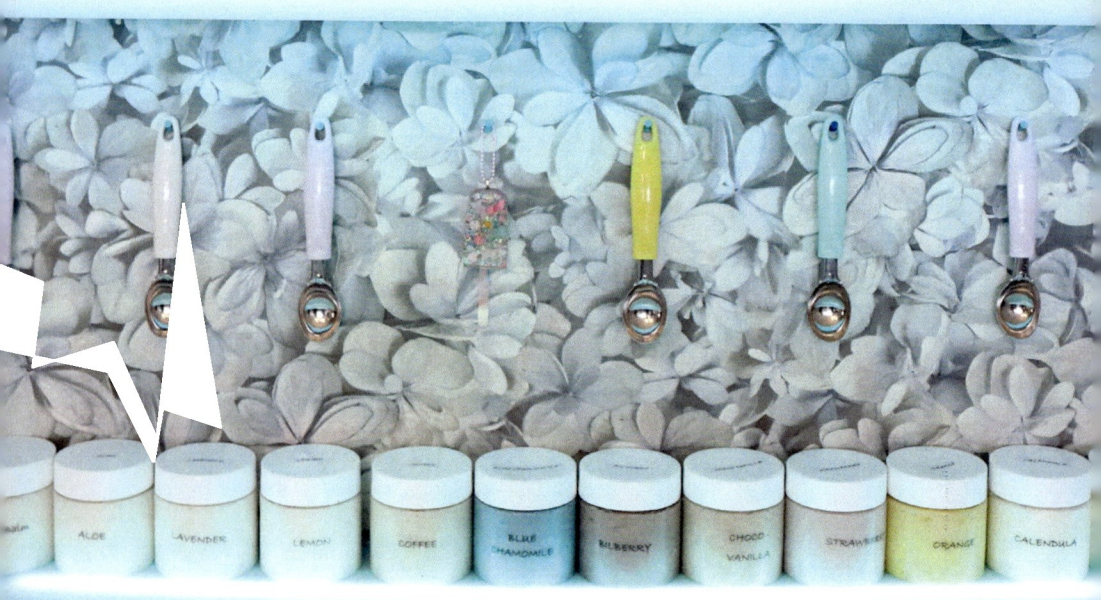

| ALOE | LAVENDER | LEMON | COFFEE | BLUE CHAMOMILE | BILBERRY | CHOCO VANILLA | STRAWBERRY | ORANGE | CALENDULA |

CREATE, BAKE AND DECORATE.

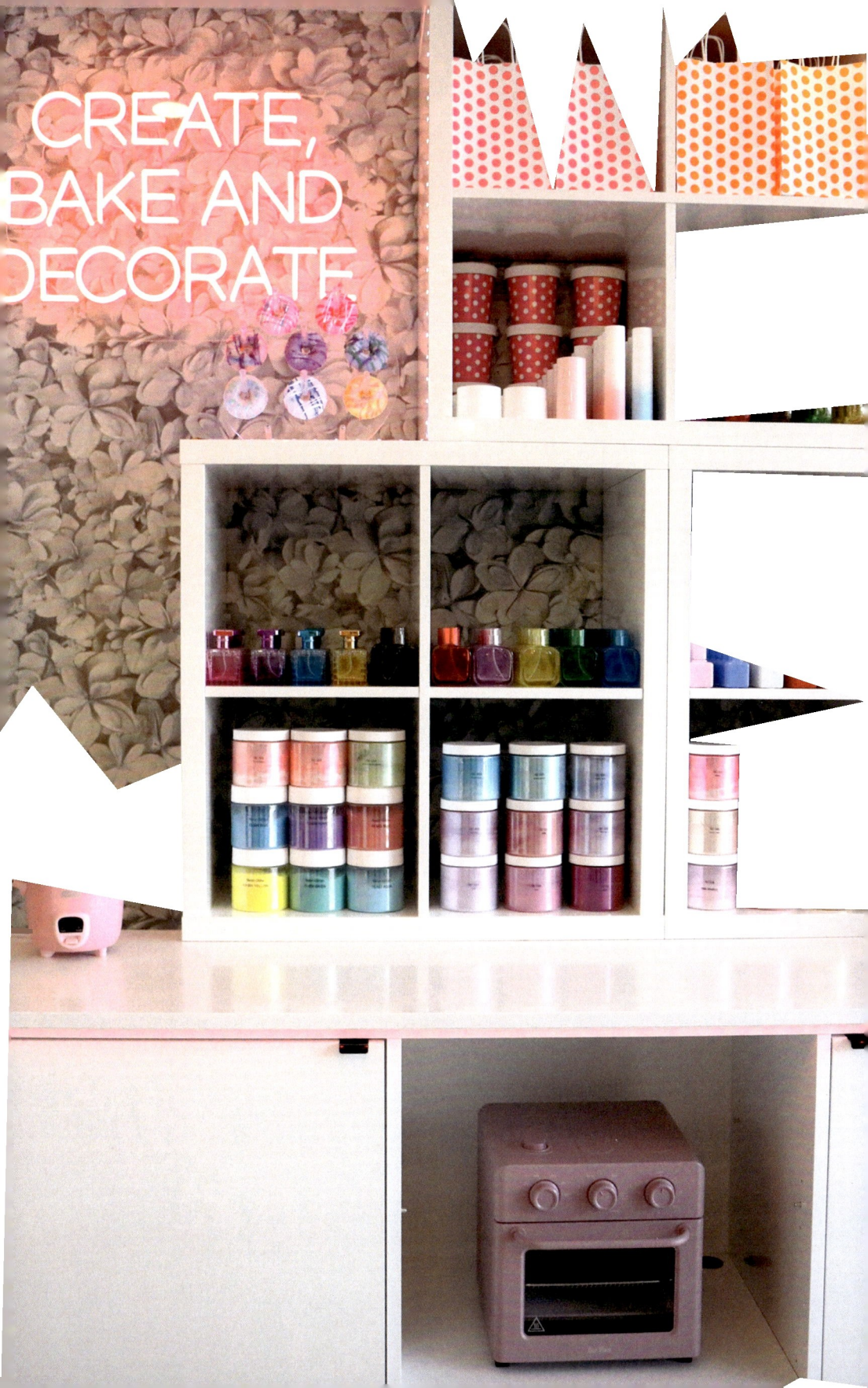